M000009202

Eat More Plants Love

RECIPES FOR A GOOD LIFE

SHARI AND DOUG SCHMIDT

Eat Plants Love Ltd

Chandler, Arizona

Copyright © 2020 by Shari and Doug Schmidt
Published by Eat Plants Love Ltd.

All rights reserved. This book, or any portion thereof,
may not be reproduced or used in any manner whatsoever
without the express written permission of the publisher
except for the use of brief quotations in a book review.

Printed in the United States of America

First Printing, 2020

ISBN 978-1-7340111-2-8

Eat Plants Love Ltd.
Chandler, Arizona
email: dkschmidt@eatplantslove.com

Ordering Information:
Quantity sales. Special discounts are available on quantity purchases by corporations, associations,
and others. For details, contact the publisher at the email address above.

Book design and photographs by Doug Schmidt

"It's never too late to change old habits."

Florence Griffith Joyner

GUIDELINES OF THE GOOD LIFE CHALLENGE

WHAT YOU WILL AVOID FOR THE 10 DAYS

All meat (beef, poultry, pork and fish)
All dairy and eggs
All highly processed foods
Oil
Smoothies, alcohol, juice and soda
added sugar and salt

WHAT YOU WILL ENJOY

All fruits, vegetables, whole grains and legumes
Greens at every meal (3-6 servings a day)
Whole grain breads
Whole grain pastas (brown rice pastas are excellent)
Mushrooms
Drink lots of water
Unsweetened tea, coffee without sweeteners and processed creamers

KEEP TO A MINIMUM

Nuts, seeds and nut butters
(limit nuts to 1 tablespoon on your oats or salads or use in sauce recipes. Do not consume nut or nut butters otherwise)
Dried Fruit
(Do not eat as a snack but use as a sweetener)
Avocados
(1/4 avocado is one serving. Limit to 1 serving a day)

Give yourself the gift of 10 days to show you how good healthy tastes and feels. After the 10 days you can use these guidelines to keep going on your plant based journey.

THE 5 GOODS

A healthy lifestyle is comprised of several components. Below are the 5 essential 'goods' for a healthy life.

GOOD FOOD

A whole food plant based diet gives your body all the nutrients it needs to not just live, but to thrive. It gives you everything you need (and more!) and can heal many of the chronic diseases plaguing us. Avoid all meat, dairy, eggs, fish and any animal products and processed foods and nourish your body with whole foods like fruit, vegetables, grains and legumes.

GOOD MOVE

You don't have to run marathons to be healthy and fit. We don't say 'exercise' daily. We say 'move' daily. Every day do some sort of movement. Do what you can depending on your level of fitness. For some it might be a walk around the block (or just to the mailbox). For others it might be going on a hike. Get out and do something you like every day. Gardening, biking , walking, running, swimming, dancing - anything to get you moving. Do something you enjoy as an activity. Get off the couch and get those joints lubricated and use those muscles! As our friend Tim Kaufman, (who lost over 200 pounds) says, "Eat plants and move your body. All ya gotta do is a little more than ya did yesterday." Note that 80% of weight loss is due to your food intake. Less than 20% is due to exercise. Keep in mind, if you have a significant amount of weight to lose, don't worry so much about movement until you lose some of that weight. It takes a lot of energy to carry around that excess weight and that, in essence, is exercise on its own. Add in more movement once you have lost some weight.

GOOD REST

Ten years ago we made a change in our bedroom. We took out the tv. At first it was a bit odd to fall asleep without noise in the background. After a few days we didn't miss it. Our sleep was deeper and more restorative. Now we talk about our bedroom as our refuge. No electronics are allowed. We keep our phones and laptops out of our bedroom. It is our place of tranquility. Lack of sleep can affect your health in a very short period of time. You need to sleep to stay healthy. Try to get 7 - 9 hours a night[1]

GOOD MOOD

Lack of sleep, anxiety and stress, all affect our mood. Diet and exercise also directly affect our mood. Eating a poor diet, one filled with animal products and processed foods, can directly affect the brain and the neuro-transmitters that help regulate your mood. It can lead to vitamin and nutrient deficiencies that also make people susceptible to mental health issues.[2] Most of the serotonin in our bodies is produced in our gut and exercise induces the production of endorphins.[3] Eating well and exercising are natural mood regulators. To

1   https://health.clevelandclinic.org/happens-body-dont-get-enough-sleep/
2   https://www.ncbi.nlm.nih.gov/pmc/articles/PMC4150387/
3   https://www.healthline.com/health/mental-health/serotonin

reduce stress you can learn how to meditate, but most importantly, learn to focus on your breathing. A long exhale can do wonders to calm the body.

GOOD FRIENDS/TRIBE

In the ground-breaking study with National Geographic and in his book, The Blue Zones, Dan Buettner discovered that there are certain regions in the world where people live long healthy lives.[1] Many of these individuals live to over 100 years of age. One of the traits common among these places is community involvement. Spend time with people that love and support you. Have those people over for dinner or meet them for a daily walk. Find people you can laugh with and enjoy their company. In the Blue Zones, people also have a purpose. They have a reason to live and feel needed. Purpose could be childcare, giving back to the community, or a job that is meaningful. Find your tribe and your purpose! Connect with other WFPB people on social media by joining the Facebook group, Eat Plants Love. Find local friends and create a monthly potluck meet-up. Finding a supportive community will help you to be successful changing to a WFPB way of life.

"We all have big changes in our lives that are more or less a second chance."

Harrison Ford

---

[1]   https://www.bluezones.com/

Change is Not Easy!

Teddy Roosevelt said, "Nothing in the world is worth having or worth doing unless it means effort, pain, difficulty... I have never in my life envied a human being who led an easy life."

Your health is worth it and your family is worth it. Trying recipes in this cookbook is that first step to a healthier you.

GOOD LIFE PROFILE: DOUG SCHMIDT

Doug, a veteran teacher, suffered a widowmaker heart attack at age 49. Not wanting to spend the rest of his life on medications, he sought answers. After finding the book, "Prevent and Reverse Heart Disease" by Dr. Caldwell Esselstyn, he changed his lifetime of eating habits. He lost 60 pounds, is off all medication, and ran his first marathon at age 58. Doug's wife Shari lost 40 pounds, ran her first half marathon at 53 and together they now lead the annual "Good Life Challenge" for teachers and staff for over 75 school districts and small businesses in New York. The challenge helps educate people about the benefits of plant based nutrition and was featured on Good Morning America. Doug and Shari manage the Facebook group, Eat Plants Love, sharing their knowledge and expertise. This is Doug and Shari's 2nd cookbook. "Eat Plants Love - Recipes for a Good Life", was their first cookbook.

Doug has a Masters in Special Education and has completed the Rouxbe Plant Based Professional Certification and is a certified CHIP and Lift project facilitator. He was formerly a professional baker who worked for one of the most prestigious grocery chains in America as their bakery trainer. Shari completed the E-Cornell course in Plant Based Nutrition and is a certified CHIP facilitator.

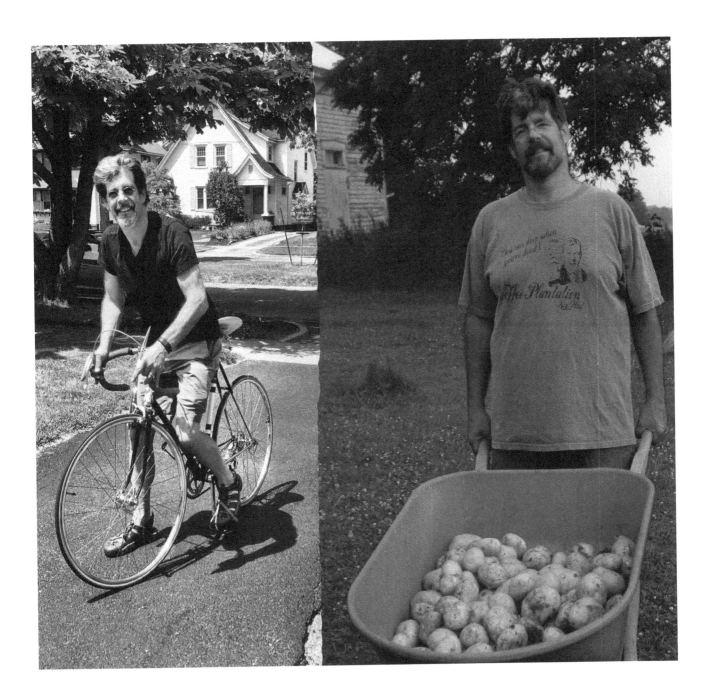

THE HEALTH CONTINUUM

Where are you on the road to health?

Think of health as a continuum. On one end is the Standard American Diet (SAD) which is one of the most nutritionally problematic ways to eat that mankind has produced. Besides the abundance of animal product consumption, many of these food-like substances are created in factories by food scientists who make hyper palatable foods, devoid of quality nutrition and typically loaded with preservatives, salt, fat and sugars. On the far other end of the spectrum is a whole plant food diet. This is the Rolls Royce of diets. It has been scientifically proven to be the best diet to eat for health and longevity. It is the only diet proven to prevent and reverse heart disease[1] and has been shown to help heal most chronic diseases like type 2 diabetes[2], autoimmune diseases[3], high cholesterol, high blood pressure and even help battle some forms of cancer.[4] There are several reasons why a whole plant diet is so powerful.

Antioxidants

A whole food plant diet is loaded with, not just vitamins and minerals, but also with antioxidants which help to prevent free radicals that cause cellular damage to your body.[5]

Phytonutrients

There are over 25,000 different phytonutrients found in plants like carotenoids, flavonoids, and resveratrol to name just a few. They help in vitamin production, immune system functioning and disease prevention. They are only found in plants.

Fiber

95% of Americans do not eat enough fiber.[6] This lack of fiber sets you up for a weakened immune system. Our gut microbiome feeds on the fiber we eat to create the beneficial bacteria that supports a healthy immune system. Fiber also only comes from plants. Just adding a protein bar with added fiber is not enough. You need intact

1   https://www.ncbi.nlm.nih.gov/pmc/articles/PMC5466936/
2   https://www.ncbi.nlm.nih.gov/pmc/articles/PMC5466941/
3   https://nutritionstudies.org/autoimmune-disease-genes-infection-environment-gut/
4   https://www.mayoclinic.org/healthy-lifestyle/nutrition-and-healthy-eating/in-depth/how-plant-based-food-helps-fight-cancer/art-20457590#:~:text=It's%20true%20plant%2Dbased%20foods,may%20protect%20cells%20from%20damage.

5   https://www.mayoclinic.org/healthy-lifestyle/nutrition-and-healthy-eating/multimedia/antioxidants/sls-20076428#:~:text=Antioxidants%20are%20substances%20that%20may,to%20tobacco%20smoke%20or%20radiation.
6   https://www.ncbi.nlm.nih.gov/pmc/articles/PMC6124841/

fiber, and different kinds, as there are two types of fiber: soluble and insoluble.

Soluble fiber dissolves in water, and includes plant pectin and gums. Insoluble fiber doesn't dissolve in water. It includes plant cellulose and hemicellulose.

Most plants contain both soluble and insoluble fiber, but in different amounts. Fiber is an important part of a healthy diet and supports many different body systems.[7]

Soluble fiber is found in oats, beans and some fruits and vegetables. Insoluble fiber—found in whole grains, fruits and vegetables, kidney beans, and bran. "The consumption of food rich in fiber also decreased the frequency of heart disease, stroke, type 2 diabetes, and CRC by 16% to 24%."[8] Fiber is only found in plants. Data from the American Gut Project has revealed that consuming more than 30 different plant-based foods on a weekly basis is associated with a widely diverse gut microbiota that helps to build a stronger immune system.[9]

Work on moving your health toward the plant eating side of the health continuum. Focus on progress, not perfection, but the ideal is to eat a whole plant diet. The closer you get to it, the healthier you will be.

7   https://www.healthline.com/health/soluble-vs-insoluble-fiber
8   https://www.mdlinx.com/article/high-fiber-diet-can-prevent-these-fatal-diseases/lfc-3720
9   https://msystems.asm.org/content/3/3/e00031-18

GOOD LIFE PROFILE: WORKING TOGETHER

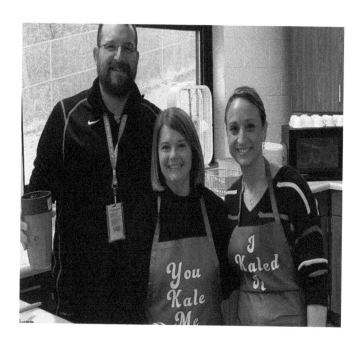

For quite a few years there have been several of us that have supported each other with workouts and running. In the last couple years, the same group has transitioned to the plant-based lifestyle. Our support for each other extends from shopping, sharing recipes and instructional cooking classes. I had my concerns starting this lifestyle having Crohn's disease, but with increased workouts and eating a plant-based diet, my symptoms have decreased. I've been through many challenges, but nothing beats where I am now.

-Robyn Monahan, RN

The Newark High School nurses and staff decided to participate in one of our challenges. Here is what they had to say about their experience:

I love, love, love that I am surrounded at work now by plant loving and eating people. My experience with vegan and vegetarian practices goes way back to my college days when I was introduced to the atrocities and the environmental degradation caused by industrial animal farming. Recently, health concerns in my immediate family brought the benefits of plant-based lifestyle front and center at the very time the first challenge was being introduced. What timing! So grateful!

-Inger Rothpearl, RN

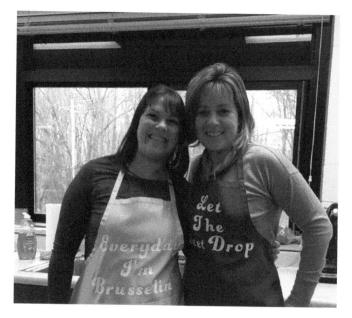

We went from an office that regularly shared cakes, donuts and cookies to an office that now shares plant based peanut butter bars, kale muffins and kale chips. It has truly been a transformative experience for us as a group and I think our ability to support and encourage one another has been such a big part of helping all of us engage in a healthier lifestyle. We all want to feel PLANT STRONG now and that's a great feeling.
–Kristin Leonard– School Psychologist

Other plant–based office members: Susan Gardner, MaryBeth Springett, Sonya Mateo, Will Bean

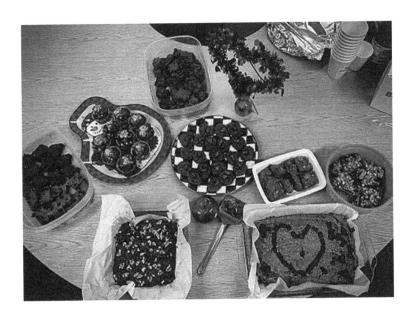

GOOD LIFE PROFILE: PATTY AND SCOTT VERBRIDGE

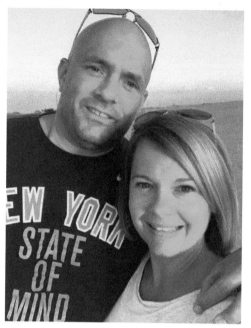 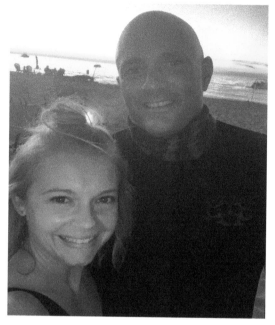

My name is Patricia Verbridge. I work with all these wonderful people who support and encourage each other. My husband Scott and I have been on the WFPB diet since 1/6/2020.

Robyn and I were planning on running a marathon in May of 2020. I knew I wanted to train on a WFPB diet. Working with Danielle, Mike, and René who had all been WFPB and were having amazing results I knew that it would be the best way to go.

In late 2019 my husband Scott and I watched some documentaries on Netflix and Amazon to help us gain some knowledge of the WFPB lifestyle. In January we set off on our new lifestyle journey. The marathon was cancelled in March, but we continued with the lifestyle. He was no longer having any pain in his shoulders, elbows and other joints (due to inflammation). We had more energy, and I was running faster and longer than ever before. The recovery time after the run was incredible. We have lost over 50lbs together and feel amazing.

I am thankful for the people I work with and that are on this same incredible health journey as I am. It is wonderful to have such a close and amazing support group here.

–Patty Verbridge– Administrative Assistant

GOOD LIFE PROFILE: DANIELLE AND MIKE MCGAVISK

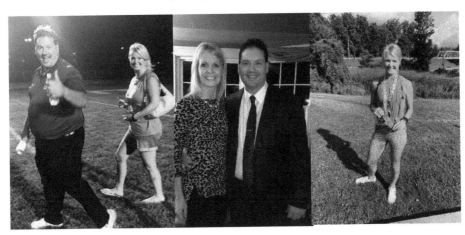

In November of 2018, my husband's mother was hospitalized. During this time, we spent almost every day visiting her in Strong Memorial Hospital. When you spend that much time in a hospital, you realize that the most important thing you have is your own health. This was also a time when the Good Life Challenge was being promoted in our school, and on top of that my husband and I were on the verge of 50. We knew people who were being diagnosed with cancer, heart disease and having strokes. I said to my husband in December...we are doing the Good Life Challenge! We had to make a change in our lifestyle, as we were both significantly overweight, our cholesterol was high and overall health was not good. We were becoming more and more sedentary and lacked the energy to be present in the lives of our three children. It was time for us.

Beginning on January 2019 it started, the kids had bets that dad wouldn't last 2 days without eating meat. Since then I have lost 52lbs, Mike has lost 80 lbs. Our blood work is PERFECT! Every issue we had is gone. We can be active with our kids and I am running 5k's with the best times of my life - at age 50!! Our increased energy and the way we feel daily, is amazing. I have become a Plant Based Coach, taught plant-based cooking classes and I try to help others make the change to a WFPB diet. I love everything about this lifestyle change and the idea of being able to live a longer healthier life with my husband and family is the ultimate reward.

-Danielle McGavisk- Director of Counseling

GOOD LIFE PROFILE: RENÉ SINICROPI

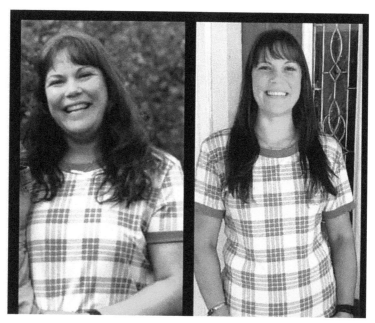

I made the decision to live a plant-based lifestyle in September of 2019. I was in a rut with my exercise and nutrition and I was the heaviest I'd ever been. I saw Danielle and Mike's journey and I knew I needed to do something different. I fully committed and lost 60 pounds in the first year. My bloodwork is incredible and the amount of energy I have has skyrocketed. I am able to keep up with my 4-year-old and show him some healthier ways to eat. We both eat the kale blueberry muffins from the Engine 2 cookbook daily and he loves to try all of the sweet treats that I make. There is not any food that I miss from my pre plant life because there is always an alternative to it. I enjoy cooking and trying new things and I am very thankful to have such a supportive office to go through this journey with. We are always sharing recipes and treats and cheering each other on. We are in this together!

-René Sinicropi- School Psychologist

"A journey of a thousand miles begins with a single step"

Lao Tzu

THE GOOD LIFE RECIPES

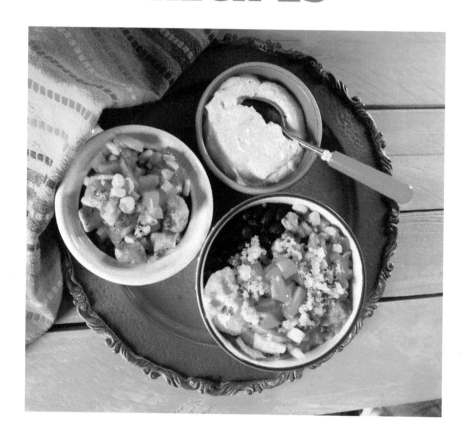

"Came from a plant, eat it;
was made in a plant, don't."

Michael Pollan

Recipes Are A Guideline

The recipes in this book should be a jumping off point. These recipes are to show you how tasty and enjoyable healthy food can be. Not all tastes are the same. We don't like cilantro, so in many recipes we replace it with parsley. Some people hate mushrooms, so don't make those recipes or take out the mushrooms. Mushrooms are extremely healthy for you. There are also many types of mushrooms available, so try out different ones. You may find one you do like. Feel free to spice things up. If you like heat in a recipe, add your favorite hot sauce or red pepper flakes.

In many of our recipes you will see common ingredients. We try to include beans and dark leafy greens or cruciferous vegetables in our recipes. These are some of the most nutritious plants. We try to eat these every day (at every meal if possible), focusing on the dark leafy greens.

Salt

Our recipes contain a minimal amount of salt. Some people have medical reasons why they cannot have salt. If you are one of those people, leave it out and use a salt substitute like Mrs. Dash™ seasonings. If you are not sensitive to salt, and are not eating a lot of processed foods, you can make our recipes as they are written. For most recipes, salt is optional and should be added to taste, as needed, before serving. Some recipes require a little salt for maximum flavor, but in most cases, we choose to salt our food minimally at the table.

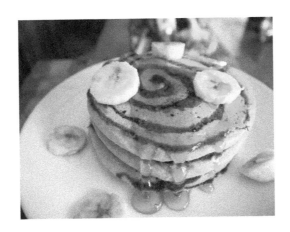

BREAKFAST IDEAS

Kayc Jo's Aquafaba Granola 22

Peachy Keen Muffins 24

Sweet Potato Breakfast Bowl 26

Anything Goes Breakfast Bowl 28

Baked Sweet Potato with Oat Crumble and Blueberries 30

Fancy Toasts 32

Papa's Pancakes 34

KAYC JO'S AQUAFABA GRANOLA

When looking online for a no-oil vegan granola recipe, I stumbled across aquafaba for the first time. Aquafaba is the liquid from canned chickpeas. This was a game changer for me. I found a recipe that was good but still had too much refined sugar in it and not enough flavor. So I kept making changes to the recipe until I found the perfect combination. I love my granola crunchy, so I use a low and slow baking method. I use the granola as a breakfast, either plain with almond milk or in an acai breakfast bowl. It's also great alone as a crunchy and satisfying snack.

Kayc Jo Cass-Northrop, Naples, NY

Liquid from 1 can of garbanzo beans (chickpeas) called Aquafaba

1 tablespoon vanilla extract

¾ cup pure maple syrup

3 cups rolled oats

1 cup chopped raw nuts (almonds, walnuts, cashews)

½ cup shredded unsweetened coconut

1 tablespoon chia seeds

2 tablespoons ground flax seed

1 teaspoon salt

2 teaspoons ground cinnamon

1. Preheat oven to 350°F.

2. Drain a can of chickpeas into a small bowl (save the chickpeas to use in another recipe).

3. Beat the aquafaba with a mixer until loose peaks form.

4. Add the vanilla and maple syrup and continue to mix until combined.

5. In a separate large bowl, mix all the dry ingredients.

6. Add the wet ingredients into the dry ingredients and mix well.

7. Spread the mixture onto a lined baking sheet.

8. Bake on the lowest rack in the oven for 30 minutes.

9. Stir and bake for another 30 minutes.

10. Continue baking and stirring every 5 minutes until the granola is brown, dry and crispy (total of 1 hour 15 minutes).

11. Remove from the oven and let cool for 10 minutes

12. Serve warm (with plant based yogurt or milk) or store in an airtight container for up to a week.

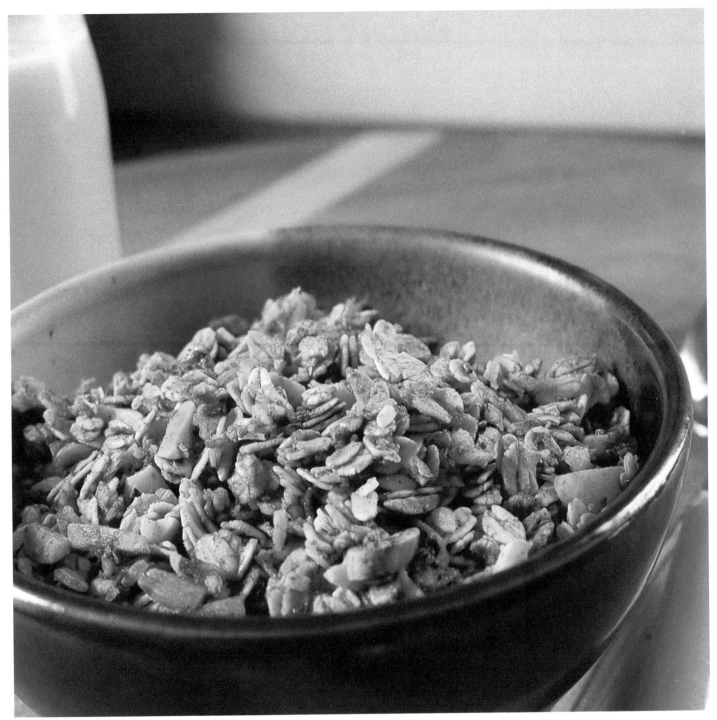

PEACHY KEEN MUFFINS

Makes 10–12 muffins

1 medium golden beet, cooked and chopped (about ¾ cup)

1 cup non-dairy milk

½ cup maple syrup

2 teaspoons almond extract

1 teaspoon lemon juice

Zest of 1 whole lemon

1 ½ cups whole wheat pastry flour

¾ cup almond meal/flour

2 teaspoons baking powder

1 teaspoon baking soda

1 teaspoon cinnamon

¼ teaspoon nutmeg

½ teaspoon salt

1 cup chopped fresh peaches

1. Preheat oven to 350°F.

2. Place beet, maple syrup, vanilla, lemon juice and lemon zest in a food processor and process until pureéd.

3. In a medium size bowl, measure out all the dry ingredients and stir until well combined.

4. Add milk and beet puree to dry ingredients and mix until no dry ingredients are seen.

5. Add chopped peaches and mix into batter.

6. Portion into silicone muffin pan (or into cupcake liners).

7. Bake at 350° for 30-35 minutes or until a toothpick comes out clean.

Note: We like using pastry flour to create a more tender muffin. All purpose whole wheat flour will work but the muffins may be a little drier and heavier.

For a plain vanilla cupcake, leave out the peaches and almond extract. Increase the vanilla extract to 2 teaspoons.

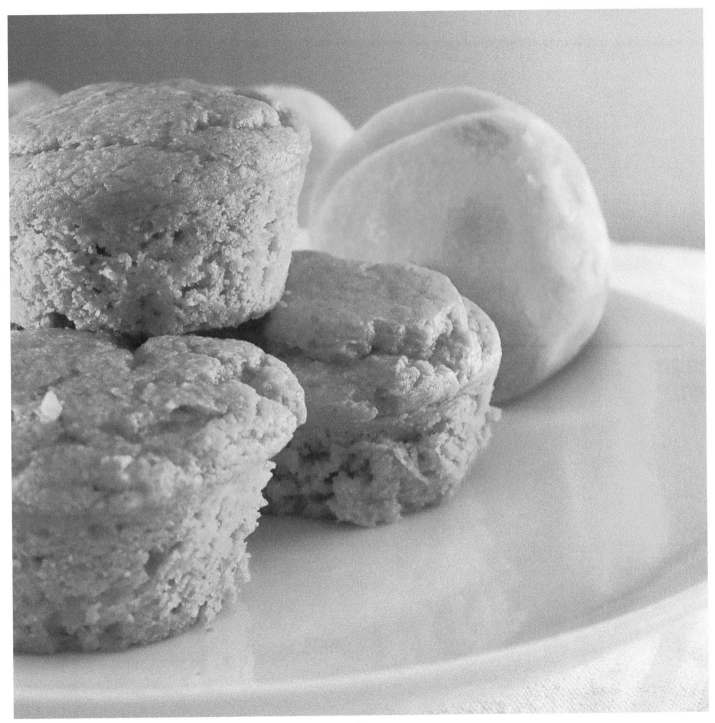

SWEET POTATO BREAKFAST BOWL

Serves 1

Lisa Roberts from Collins, NY said that a unique coffee shop in Springville, NY had something similar on their menu but it was overly sweetened with brown sugar. She figured she could make it less sweet and add anything she wanted to it and have it for breakfast.

1 sweet potato

2 tablespoons pecans

1 tablespoon maple syrup

1 tablespoon raisins

1 tablespoon chia seeds

Cinnamon to taste

Non-dairy milk

1. Bake or microwave a sweet potato.

2. Top with pecans, maple syrup, raisins, chia seeds.

3. Sprinkle with cinnamon and a splash of non-dairy milk.

Note: Change up the toppings to your liking. Use walnuts or almonds. Try it with green apples or craisins.

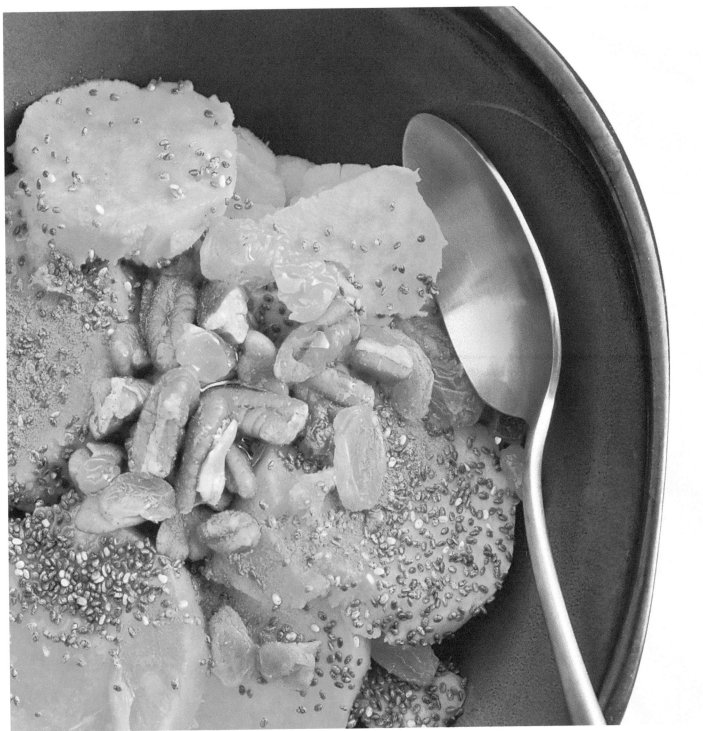

ANYTHING GOES BREAKFAST BOWL

Serves 3 – 4

Cassie Montemarano submitted this delicious recipe. She makes this to use up ingredients she has on hand at the end of the week. It is so filling, we had it for dinner one night. Add some beans to make it a complete meal.

1 yellow potato, diced

1 red potato, diced

1 sweet potato, diced

Dash of cayenne pepper

¼ teaspoon turmeric

¼ teaspoon garlic powder

½ cup diced onions

3 garlic cloves, minced

½ - 1 cup mushrooms, sliced

1 pepper, diced

½ cup salsa

2 cups spinach

2 cups kale, chopped

Salt and pepper to taste

Hot sauce (optional)

1 avocado, sliced

1. In a large skillet, add potatoes, cayenne pepper, turmeric and garlic powder and sauté for about 5 minutes, adding 1 - 2 tablespoons of water at a time to prevent sticking.

2. Add onions and garlic and sauté for 5 minutes more.

3. Add mushrooms and pepper and sauté for another 5 minutes.

4. Add salsa, spinach and kale and sauté until the potatoes are tender.

5. Season with salt and pepper,

6. Place in a bowl, season with hot sauce and top with sliced avocado.

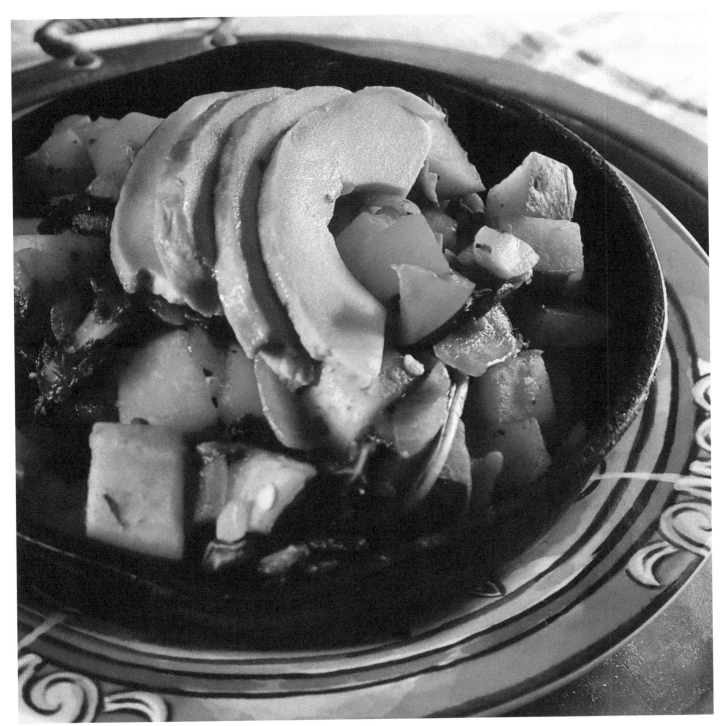

BAKED SWEET POTATO WITH OAT CRUMBLE AND BLUEBERRIES

Serves 2

2 large sweet potatoes

½ cup rolled oats

¼ cup nuts (we like a sliced almond/walnut combination)

½ tsp ground flax seed

½ teaspoon cinnamon

Pinch of salt

3 tablespoons maple syrup

1 cup fresh blueberries

1. Preheat the oven to 400°F.

2. Wash the potatoes and pierce with a fork several times and place on a lined baking sheet. Bake for about 45 - 50 minutes. Set aside to cool.

3. Lower the oven temperature to 350 degrees.

4. Mix the oats, nuts, flax seed, cinnamon and salt in a small bowl. Add in the maple syrup and mix until everything is coated.

5. Spread on a lined cookie sheet and bake for 15-20 minutes, stirring halfway.

6. Split the sweet potato lengthwise and top with the oat/nut mix.

7. Top with blueberries and serve.

Note: You can use Kayc Jo's Aquafaba Granola (Page 22) instead of the oat crumble mixture. You can also microwave the sweet potatoes to save time, but we think they are more flavorful baked.

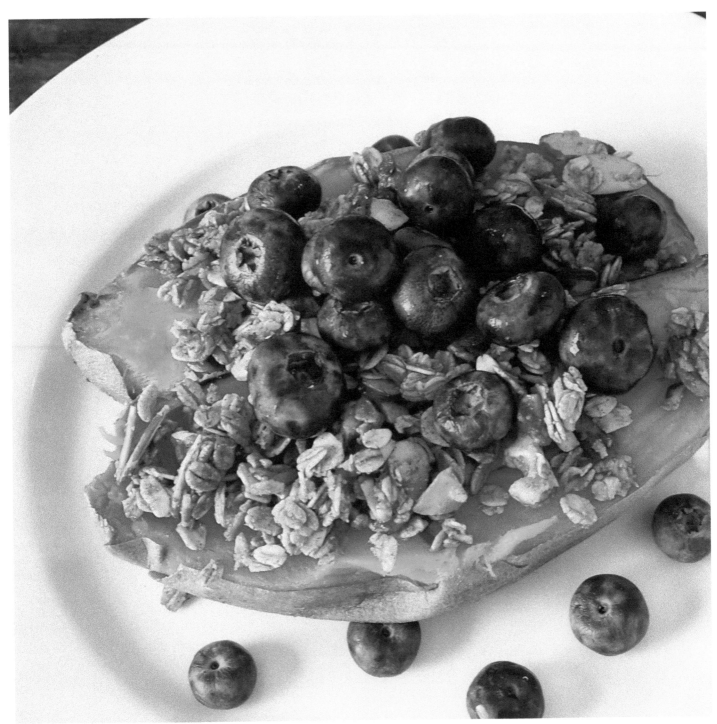

FANCY TOASTS

When visiting our son in San Francisco, he took us to a wonderful bakery called 'The Mill' for breakfast. They made wonderful toasts on inch thick sourdough bread. These are our versions with a healthy bent.

AVOCADO ON TRAILHEAD BREAD

(page 108)

Hummus

Sliced avocado

Sliced red onion

Sprouts

Flaked salt

BERRYGASM ON PEANUT BUTTER BREAD

(page 106)

Peanut butter

All fruit jam with no added sugar

Berries of choice

The secret is to make the slices nice and thick so they can hold all the ingredients without bending.

HUMMUS, TOMATO AND CUKES ON SHARI'S OATMEAL BREAD

(page 104)

Canellinni hummus (page 98)

Sliced tomatoes

Sliced cucumbers

Minced red onion

Toast your bread of choice, add toppings and create your own 'Fancy Toasts'!

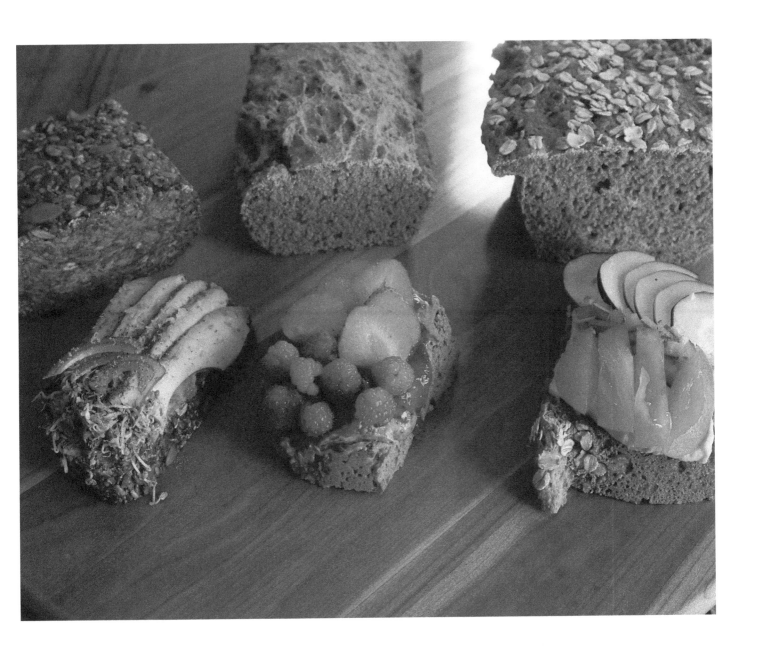

PAPA'S PANCAKES

Grandchild approved, these fluffy pancakes are the perfect breakfast for the weekend.

Makes 6–8 large pancakes

1 ½ cups white whole wheat flour

½ cup oat flour

2 tablespoons baking powder

1 teaspoon salt

2 cups non-dairy milk

2 tablespoons apple cider vinegar

4 tablespoons maple syrup

2 teaspoons vanilla

maple syrup and bananas to serve (or other fruit, like berries or peaches)

1. Place all dry ingredients into a large bowl. Stir until well combined, being careful that none of the baking powder is clumped in the mixture.

2. In a separate bowl, combine all the liquid ingredients. Stir until mixed well. Let the liquid sit until it thickens (5 minutes).

3. Mix the two mixtures together until fully blended.

4. Use a half cup measure for portioning out the pancakes onto a hot, nonstick griddle. We cook it on a griddle that is 400• F for 2½ - 3 minutes per side.

Notes:

· All the liquids should be at room temperature. This helps to prevent raw spots in the center of the pancake.

· We like to use either whole wheat pastry flour or white whole wheat flour. Pastry flour will make a more tender pancake.

· If the batter is too thin, add a quarter cup more whole wheat flour. If it is too thick, add a little more non-dairy milk.

· If you don't have an electric griddle to determine the correct temperature, put a drop of water onto the skillet. It should bubble and dance for about 3 seconds until it evaporates.

· If making blueberry pancakes, use frozen wild blueberries as they have more flavor. Drop them in the batter on the griddle so you can control how many blueberries are in each one. Press them in lightly.

· We like to top ours with fresh berries and sliced banana but get creative and top them with whatever fruit you like.

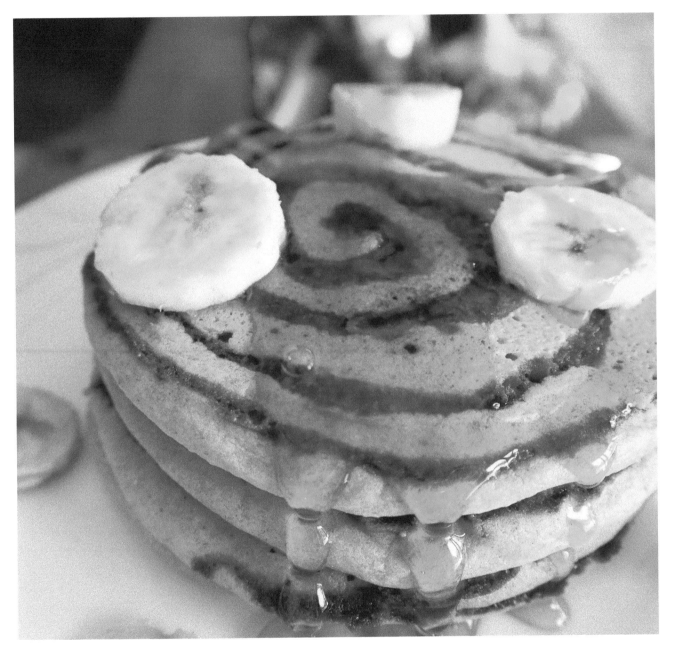

Try making cinnamon roll pancakes! Combine ½ cup of the batter with 1½ tablespoons cinnamon and 1 teaspoon cocoa. Stir until well combined. Place into a squeeze bottle and squeeze a swirl (or any design) into your pancakes as they cook.

GOOD LIFE PROFILE: CASSIE MONTEMARANO

"I grew up in a traditional meat and potatoes home also eating many processed foods. I had once done a 10 day challenge based on the Engine 2 guidelines and stuck with it a little longer than the challenge, but ultimately had gone back to former eating habits. I began incorporating more plant based meals and exercising regularly, but still had meat and dairy. After an unfortunate event at a doctor's office (for a knee injury) that resulted in my losing consciousness, falling and hitting my head, a broken nose and severe concussion, I was forced to stop exercising for an extensive period of time. Shortly after that, I was laid off from my job for the following school year. During the period of recovering from my concussion and finding my new dream job, I had gained a great deal of weight. In the fall of that school year, I knew that I needed to make a permanent lifestyle change. In December, I participated in a biometric screening to get a baseline reading of my health. My cholesterol and triglycerides needed improvement and I knew from participating in the last challenge how phenomenally my numbers had improved a few years prior. In January, I committed to beginning a whole food plant based life style and avoiding oils. I also joined the wellness challenge led by Doug and Shari Schmidt later that winter. Doug and Shari Schmidt's first cookbook, Eat Plants Love, helped me to fall in love with cooking tasty meals and their Facebook group has been a huge resource for great recipes and support from like-minded people! My husband has joined me on this journey and has also had great success. After 138 days I am down 50 pounds and my journey isn't over yet! More importantly I FEEL great, strong and healthy. I am back to being so much more active engaging in activities such as hiking and running. This has become a lifestyle change and way of life. I have made this commitment to eat this way and have said goodbye to old habits for good. Food truly is medicine and can heal a very unhealthy body."

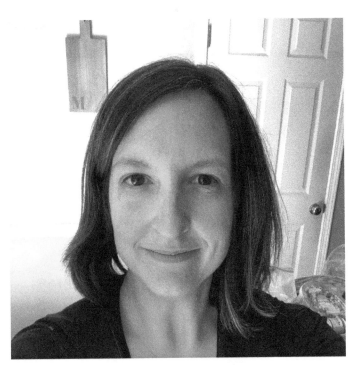

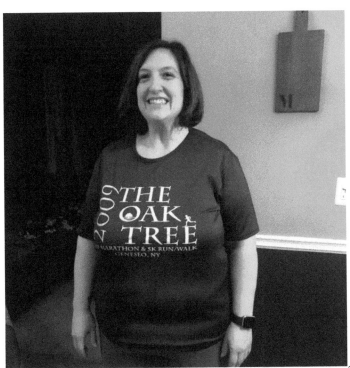

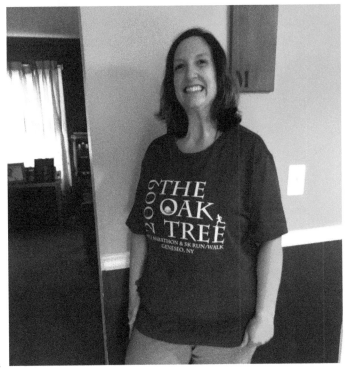

"It's not about perfect. It's about effort. And when you bring that effort every single day, that's where transformation happens."

Jillian Michaels

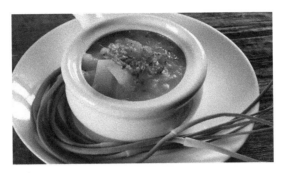

SOUPS, SALADS, SIDES AND SUCH

ROASTED CORN AND POTATO CHOWDER

Doug's mother was Pennsylvania Dutch and made a traditional dish called corn pie. This is, by far, a healthier version, without the crust.

Serves 4

3 ½ cups frozen corn, thawed (divided)

1 onion, diced

2 celery ribs, finely chopped

1 cup shiitake mushrooms, sliced

4 sprigs fresh thyme

3 cups low sodium vegetable broth

1 pound of potatoes, chopped into bite size pieces (we like Yukon gold)

2 cups fresh baby spinach

1 cup non-dairy milk

½ cup nutritional yeast

Salt and pepper to taste

1. In a large frying pan, take 2 cups of corn and dry sauté 1 cup at a time until corn starts to brown. Set aside.

2. Sauté the onion, mushrooms and celery in a 4 qt soup pot until the onions are soft.

3. Add thyme, broth and potatoes. Cook until potatoes are soft (about 20-25 minutes).

4. Remove thyme sprigs.

5. Add roasted corn and spinach.

6. Take the other 1 ½ cups of corn and the non-dairy milk and purée in a blender or food processor. Add to the soup.

7. Stir in the nutritional yeast and spinach.

8. Once spinach has wilted, taste and season with salt and pepper.

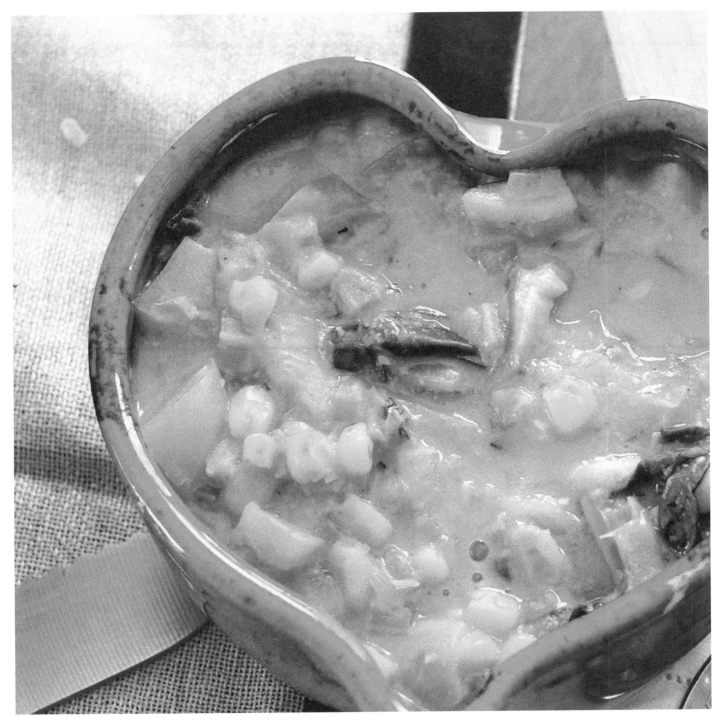

INSTANT POT CHOLENT (BEAN STEW)

Serves 8

1 pound of dried beans (we like to use a kidney, cannellini and chickpeas combination but any combination will work)

2 large onions, chopped

Pinch of baking soda

½ cup barley

4 - 5 medium yellow potatoes, ½ inch cubed (peeled if desired)

1 (14.5 oz.) can diced tomatoes

1 cup cremini mushrooms, sliced

1 teaspoon garlic powder

2 cups vegetable broth

4 cups water

2 tablespoons EPL Onion Soup mix (page 83)

2 teaspoons Marmite™

2 teaspoons low sodium soy sauce

½ cup water

1. Soak beans overnight. Rinse and drain.

2. Set Instant Pot to Sauté. Sauté onions with baking soda until soft and translucent.

3. Add in barley, potatoes, tomatoes, mushrooms, garlic powder, vegetable broth and water.

4. Combine the soup mix with marmite, soy sauce and water and pour into the Instant Pot.

5. Set Instant Pot to Manual, high pressure, for 25 minutes. Let the pressure release naturally. The longer it sits, the better the flavor.

Note: Traditionally, cholent is a Jewish stew that is set on the stove on Friday evenings to make it possible to eat something hot on the Sabbath for lunch. This recipe has all the flavor without the unhealthy ingredients. It can be made on the stovetop, but make sure it is a low flame to prevent burning. Cook overnight on low. This can also be made in a crock pot. Simply sauté the onions, add in the rest and cook for 8 hours on low.

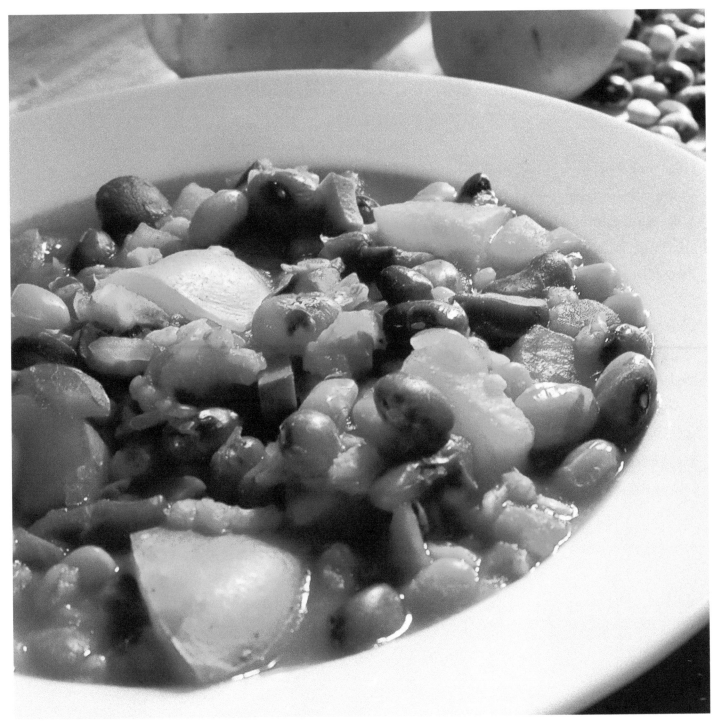

EASY CHEEZY POTATO BROCCOLI SOUP

Serves 4

1 large onion, chopped

3 stalks celery, chopped

4 cups peeled potatoes, diced

1 quart vegetable broth (4 cups)

2 ½ cups broccoli, chopped

¼ cup cornstarch

1 cup non-dairy milk

1 cup Melissa's Cheez Sauce (Page 96)

½ teaspoon smoked paprika

salt to taste

¼ teaspoon pepper

fresh parsley, chopped

1. In a 4 quart pot, sauté onion and celery until soft.

2. Add the potatoes and the vegetable broth. Set a timer for 20 minutes. Bring to a boil and then reduce to a simmer until the time runs out and potatoes are tender.

3. While potatoes are simmering, steam the broccoli for 5 minutes, remove from heat and cool under running cold water.

4. Once potatoes are tender, in a small bowl, mix the non-dairy milk and cornstarch together and stir into the soup.

5. Add broccoli, cheez sauce, smoked paprika, salt and pepper. Cook for 2 minutes more.

6. Serve with fresh chopped parsley on top.

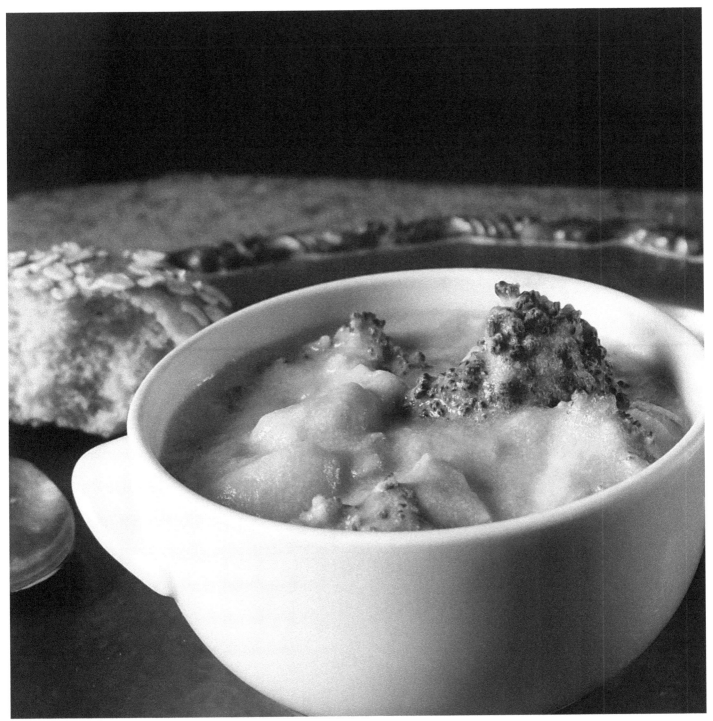

ULTIMATE WFPB CHILI

Serves 6- 8

*Nick Kline submitted this amazing chili that is chock-full of
healthy, colorful vegetables. Super satisfying! Serve with a salad
and some corn bread for a complete, delicious meal.*

½ cup onion, chopped
2 cloves garlic, minced
1 cup celery, diced
1 cup carrots, diced
2 cups sweet potato, peeled and cubed
2 cups butternut squash, peeled and cubed
1 cup bell pepper, seeded and cubed
1 (14.5 oz.) can diced tomatoes (fire roasted)
¾ cup salsa
4 cups vegetable broth
1 teaspoon salt
½ teaspoon pepper
1 bay leaf
1 ½ tablespoon chili powder
1 teaspoon ground cumin
½ teaspoon dried oregano
¼ teaspoon smoked paprika
¼ teaspoon coriander
¼ teaspoon red pepper flakes
1 teaspoon dried parsley
1 cup zucchini, chopped
2 cups kale, chopped
2 cups spinach, chopped
4 tablespoons lime juice
1 cup frozen corn
1 (15 oz.) can black beans, drained and rinsed
1 (15 oz.) can kidney beans, drained and rinsed
½ cup chopped fresh cilantro (or parsley)

1. In a large stock pot or dutch oven over medium heat, sauté onion, garlic and celery. Cook, stirring frequently, until the onion has softened and turned translucent (about 5 minutes).

2. Stir in carrots, sweet potato, butternut squash, bell pepper, tomatoes, and salsa. Cook for another 5-10 minutes.

3. Add vegetable broth. Add seasonings and spices (salt through parsley). Increase heat to medium-high and bring to a boil. Reduce heat to medium-low, cover, and simmer for 10 minutes. Stir the chili occasionally to keep it from sticking.

4. Add zucchini. Simmer for about 5-10 more minutes.

5. Stir in kale, spinach, lime juice, corn, beans, and cilantro. Cook until the potatoes are tender but not mushy (about 5 minutes).

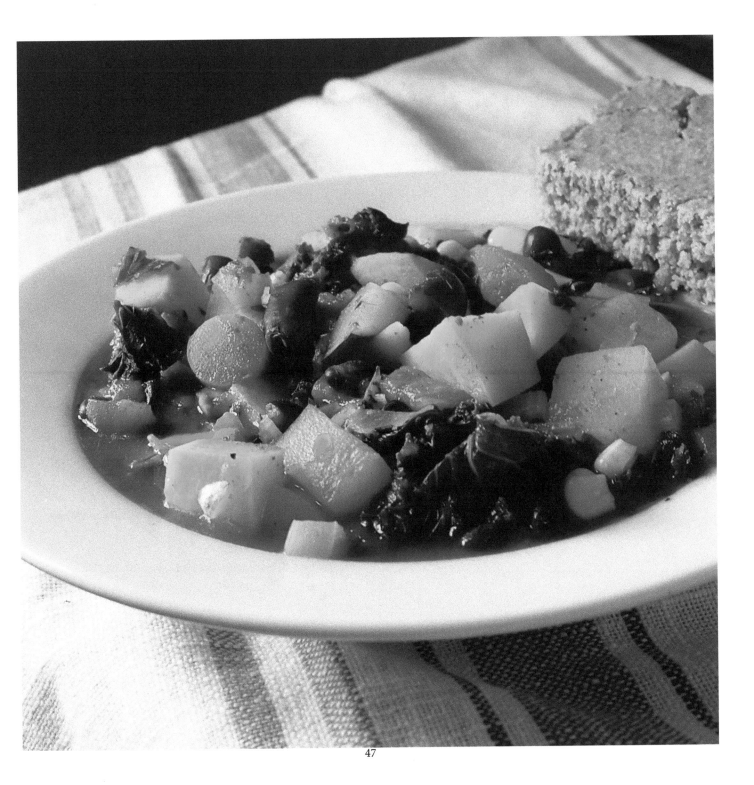

SWEET POTATO AND ONION BISQUE

Serves 8

2 quarts low sodium vegetable broth

5 large sweet onions, thinly sliced

1 ½ tablespoons maple syrup

4 medium sweet potatoes, peeled and cubed

½ teaspoon ground nutmeg

½ teaspoon ground allspice

4 sprigs fresh thyme (or 1 teaspoon dried thyme)

½ teaspoon salt

½ teaspoon ground pepper

1. In a large pot over medium-high heat, sauté onions in 2 tablespoons broth for about 10 minutes or until starting to brown.

2. Add in the maple syrup and stir for another 3 minutes.

3. Add in the rest of the broth and the sweet potatoes and seasonings and bring to a boil.

4. Reduce the heat to low and continue to simmer, uncovered, for another 20 minutes or until the sweet potato cubes are cooked through.

5. Remove the thyme sprigs (if using) and pureé the soup using an immersion blender (or pour into a blender in batches). Leave some chunks if you like your bisque that way.

6. Adjust the seasonings to taste and serve.

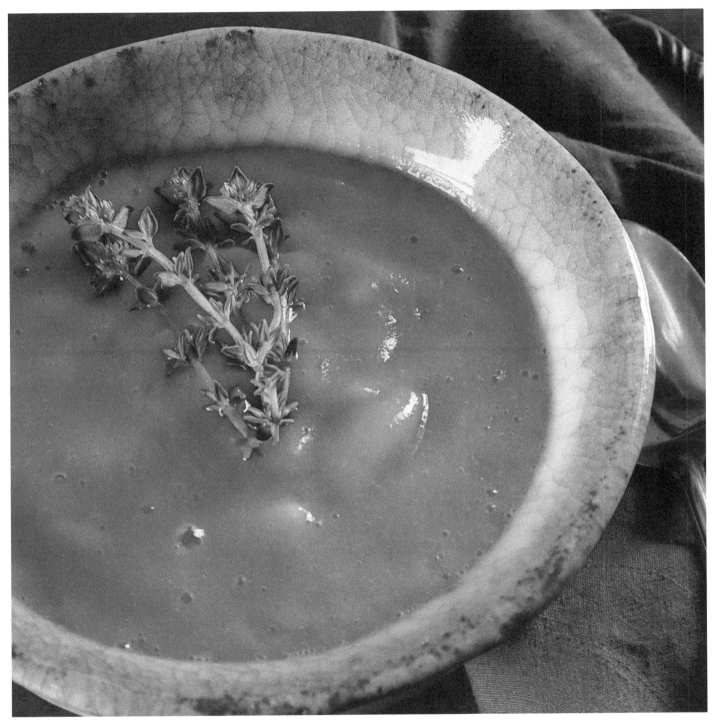

FOUR LILY SOUP

Serves 4

1 large yellow onion, sliced

½ cup garlic scapes or scallions, minced

2 leeks, sliced thinly (just the white part)

2 cloves garlic, minced

2 celery stalks, diced

2 cups vegetable stock or broth

4 medium potatoes, cubed

1 tablespoon dried rosemary

2 cups non-dairy milk

Salt and pepper to taste

1. Place the onion, garlic scapes, leeks and garlic into a 4 qt (or larger) soup pot. Cook on low heat, sweating the onions to release their moisture and soften. Cook for about 10 minutes.

2. Add celery and stock and increase the heat to bring to a boil.

3. Add potatoes, rosemary and non-dairy milk.

4. Cover and simmer (on low) until potatoes are cooked through (about 20 minutes).

5. Puree half (use an immersion blender or put half into a blender) to make it creamier.

6. Garnish with chopped scallions or Frizzled Leeks.

FRIZZLED LEEKS

When we buy leeks most recipes call for one, but our grocer only sells them in bunches of 2 or 3. What to do with extra leeks? Frizzle them. Normally, these are fried in oil. We like our healthier version. These are great on top of burgers and soups.

Preheat the oven to 350°F.
Slice leeks (just the white) into very thin slices.
Sauté them in a dry skillet until they start to brown and soften.
Transfer them to the oven and bake at 350°F until nice and crispy, about 10 minutes. Store at room temperature in a covered container.

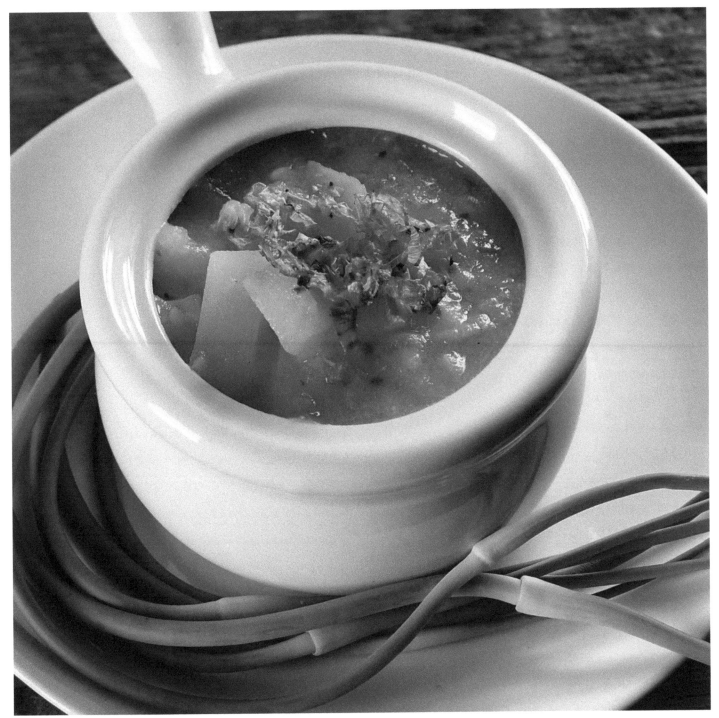

PEANUT STEW

Serves 4

Warm and nourishing. Perfect for a cold fall or winter day.

2 medium onions, chopped

2 stalks of celery, chopped

2 carrots, chopped

1 roasted red pepper, chopped

6 cloves of garlic, minced

1 tablespoon ground cumin

1 sweet potato, cut into ½ inch cubes

2 cups vegetable broth or water (½ cup reserved)

2 tablespoons mushroom powder

1 (28 oz.) can fire roasted tomatoes

1 (15 oz.) can of chickpeas, drained and rinsed

½ cup peanut butter (only peanuts, no oil added)

½ small can tomato paste

2 cups chopped kale

Salt and pepper to taste

1. In a medium size pot, sauté the onions, celery and carrots until the onions are soft.

2. Add the roasted red pepper, garlic and cumin. Sauté for another 1-2 minutes.

3. Add the sweet potato and the broth/water, reserving ½ cup of liquid to mix with the peanut butter and tomato paste.

4. Stir in the mushroom powder, fire roasted tomatoes, and chickpeas and bring to a boil, then lower to a simmer.

5. Cook until the sweet potatoes are tender.

6. Mix the peanut butter, reserved liquid and tomato paste together and add to the stew.

7. Add the kale and cook until the kale wilts. Season with salt and pepper and serve alone or over a bed of rice or any cooked whole grain.

Note: You can make your own mushroom powder by pulverizing dried mushrooms in a blender.

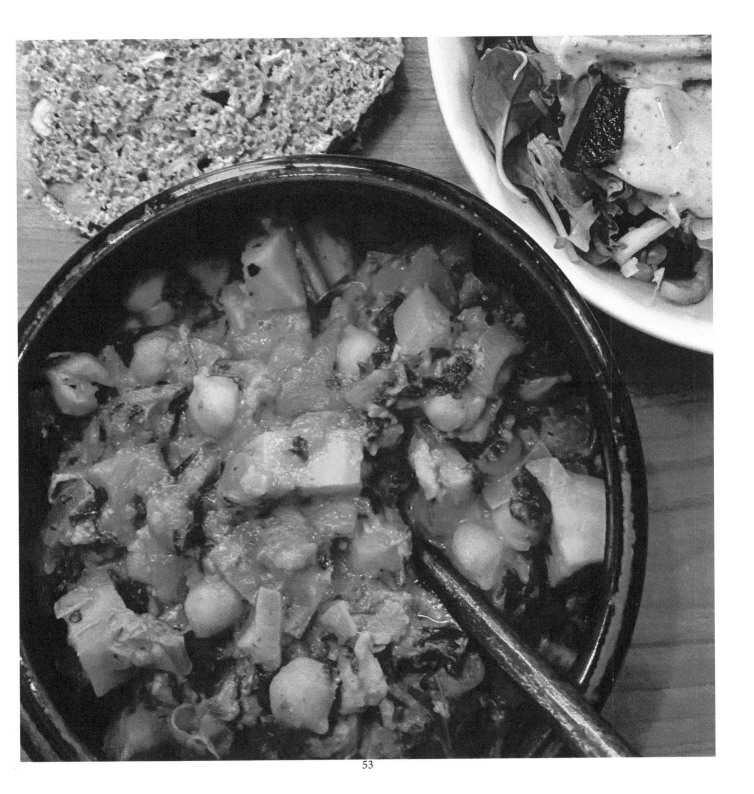

GINNY'S INSTANT POT MINESTRONE SOUP

This recipe was submitted by Ginny Trimble from western NY.
She likes to serve this with a slice of crusty bread.

1 cup diced onion

1 cup diced celery

2 large carrots, sliced or diced

6 cups low sodium vegetable broth (plus 1 extra if needed)

1 zucchini quartered and sliced in small chunks

1 (15 oz.) can cannellini or kidney beans, drained and rinsed

2 cups thinly sliced/shredded cabbage

1 (28oz.) can diced tomatoes

2 tablespoons tomato paste

2 cups diced potatoes

2 cups chopped frozen or fresh spinach

2 teaspoons (or more) minced garlic

¾ teaspoon oregano

2 bay leaves

½ cup nutritional yeast

1 tablespoon dried parsley

1 teaspoon sea salt

½ teaspoon black pepper

1 cup uncooked whole grain pasta

1 tablespoon maple syrup (optional)

1. Set the Instant Pot to Sauté. When it is hot, add onions, celery and carrots. Sauté for 5 minutes. Add garlic and sauté one minute more. Add a splash of water if it starts to stick.

2. Add the rest of the ingredients except for the extra vegetable broth (zucchini, beans, cabbage, tomatoes, tomato paste, potatoes, spinach, garlic, oregano, bay leaves, nutritional yeast, parsley, salt, pepper, pasta and maple syrup if using).

3. Hit cancel on your Instant Pot. Put the lid on and select Manual for 4 minutes. When it stops, press cancel and manually release the pressure.

4. Remove the lid and stir in some extra vegetable broth to cool it or if it is too thick and remove the bay leaves.

Note: This recipe uses elbow shaped pasta. If you are using thicker pasta, you might want to increase the cooking time to 5 or 6 minutes.

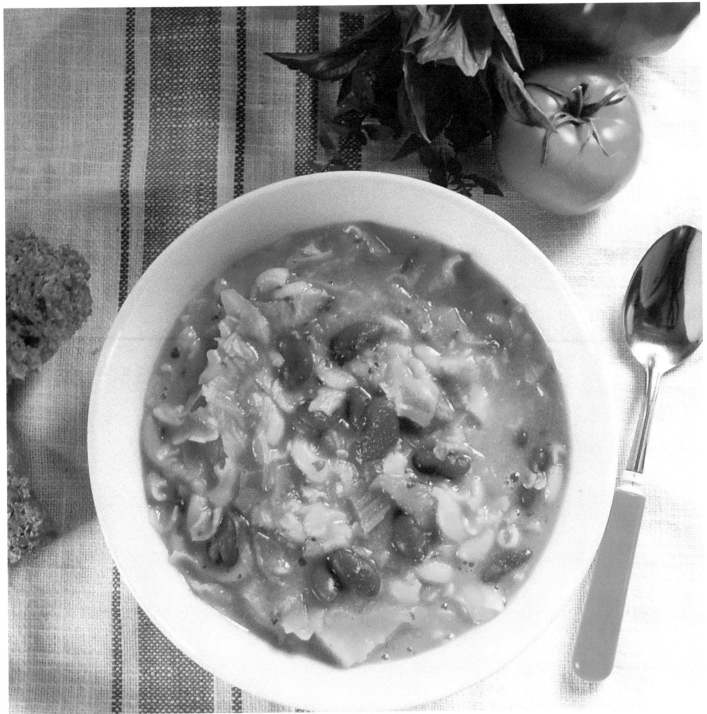

SPINACH QUINOA SALAD WITH STRAWBERRY BASIL DRESSING

Serves 4

Laurie Hansen from Hendersonville, NC submitted this recipe for a refreshing summer salad. The dressing is amazing!

2 cups cooked quinoa, cooled

8 cups fresh spinach

2 - 4 cups fresh strawberries, sliced

4 tablespoons walnuts, chopped

FOR THE DRESSING:

1 ½ cups sliced fresh strawberries

¼ cup basil leaves

2 tablespoons lemon juice

2 tablespoons apple cider vinegar

2 tablespoons balsamic vinegar

4 tablespoons maple syrup

1. Toss quinoa with spinach, strawberries and walnuts.

2. Combine the dressing ingredients in a blender and blend until smooth. Add water as needed to thin to desired consistency.

3. Divide the salad into 4 portions and drizzle with the dressing and serve.

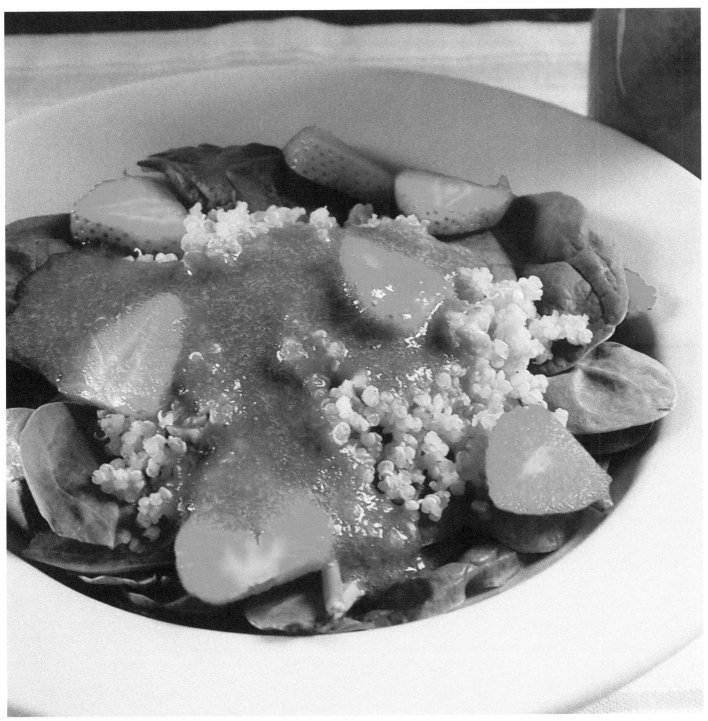

ELLEN'S BEET SALAD

Makes about 4 cups

One day while thinking about my greens intake, I thought 'why not a beet salad?', so I whipped this up using a version of the EPL Vinaigrette (which is my new favorite dressing of all time!) I love this over a bed of greens to give it a bit of a crunch!

Ellen J Monroe

3 cups beets, boiled whole then diced

1 cup red onion, diced

1 ½ cups celery, diced

EPL Vinaigrette (page 94)

1. Combine beets, onion and celery in a large bowl.

2. Make the EPL Vinaigrette dressing.

3. Pour half of the dressing over the beet mixture and stir.

Serve chilled.

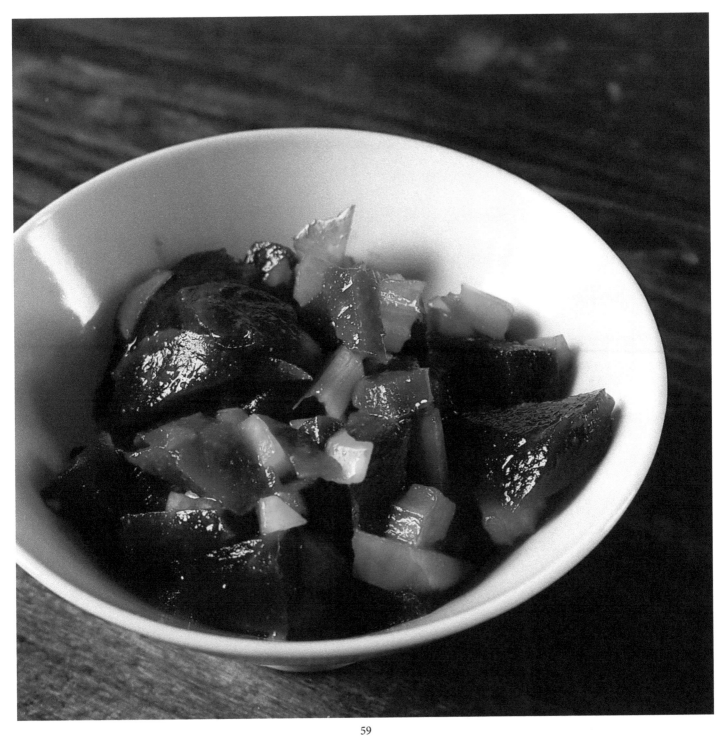

NOT CHIKEN SALAD

Serves 4

Do you miss chicken salad? You don't have to anymore.

½ bag of Butler Soy Curls™

1 batch of Tofu Mayonnaise (page 95)

1 stalk of celery, chopped (about ⅓ cup)

⅓ cup chopped red onion

1 teaspoon garlic powder

1 teaspoon onion powder

1 teaspoon poultry seasoning

Salt and pepper to taste

1. Preheat the oven to 400° F.

2. Rehydrate the soy curls in water for 10 minutes. Drain. Toss with garlic powder, onion powder, poultry seasoning, salt and pepper,.

3. Bake the soy curls for 15 minutes.

4. Place the cooled soy curls into a food processor and pulse into small bits (but not minced).

5. In a large bowl, stir the soy curls and the rest of the ingredients, adding just enough Tofu Mayonnaise to coat.

6. Keep refrigerated until ready to use.

7. Serve in a salad or on a whole grain roll with greens and a slice of tomato.

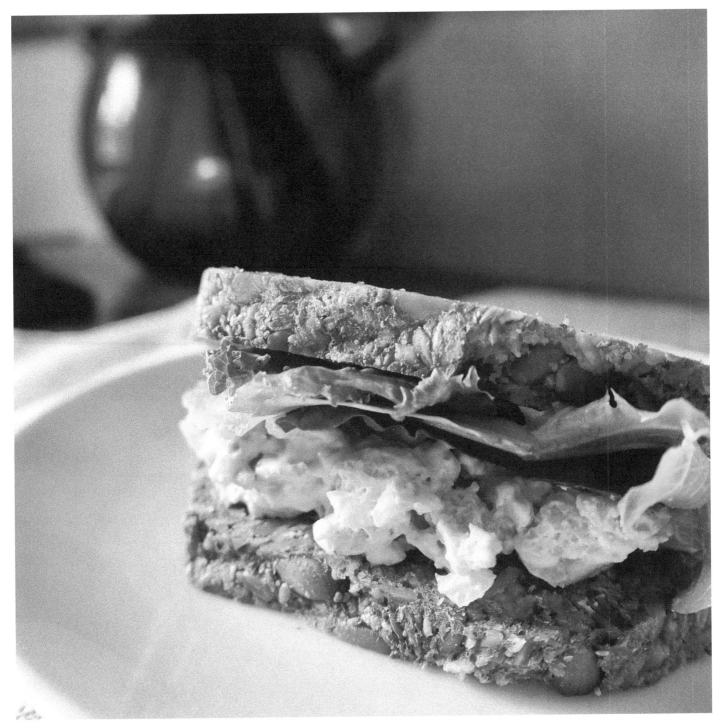

SWEET SLAW

Serves 4

1 lb bag slaw mix

10 oz bag shredded red cabbage

3 scallions, chopped

½ - ¾ cup French Dressing (Page 92)

1. Combine all ingredients in a bowl. Mix until coated evenly.

2. Serve along with (or on top of) Barbecue Sliders (Page 126).

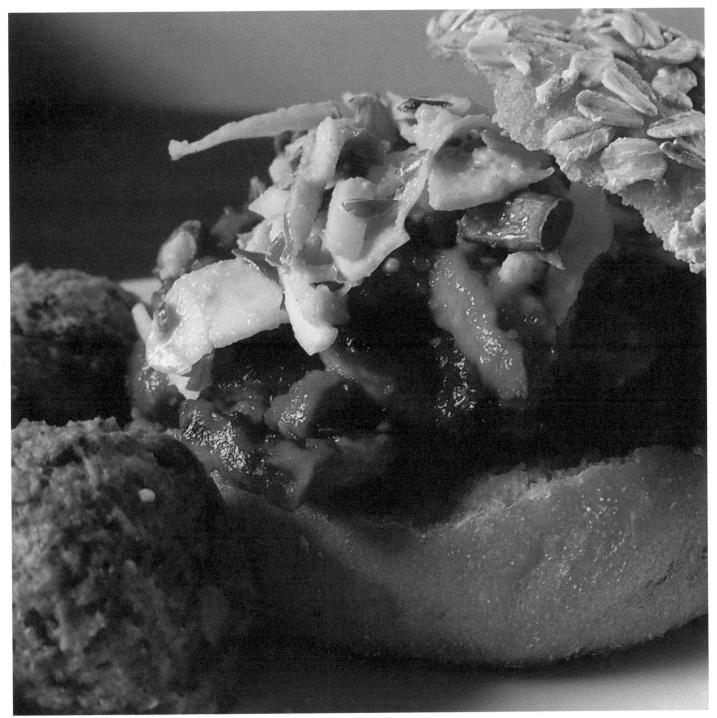

'PICKLED' CARROTS

3 carrots, cut into matchsticks or grated on a mandolin
salt
½ cup rice vinegar
¼ cup cooking wine
3 tablespoons maple syrup
3 tablespoons coconut aminos
1 tablespoon white sesame seeds
1 tablespoon black sesame seeds

1. Boil water in a medium pot and add about a heaped teaspoon of salt. Add in the carrots to blanch. Count to 10. Remove carrots, rinse in ice cold water and drain.

2. In a large bowl, mix the rice vinegar, wine, maple syrup and coconut aminos.

3. Toss the carrots into the bowl with the sauce and mix well.

4. Add sesame seeds and toss again.

5. Store in a jar and keep refrigerated. It stays crunchy and fresh for months. Add to Asian dishes or salads.

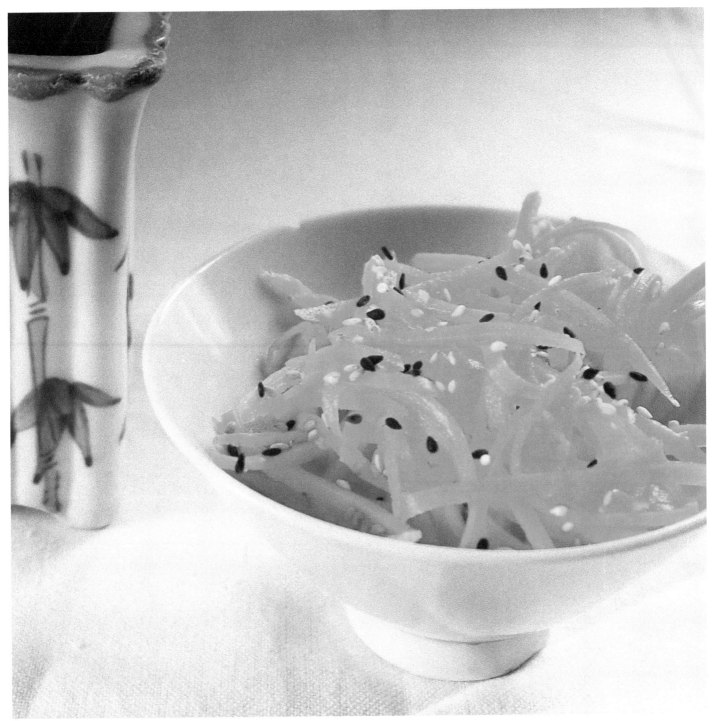

RAINBOW FARRO SALAD

Makes 2 main dishes or 4 sides

At the end of the first week of the Good Life Challenge, I had some leftover farro in the fridge and a little of this-and-that produce to use up when I was the only one home. This is what resulted! –
Haley Bibee, Sterling, NY

3 cups cooked farro, cooled

1 cup shredded red cabbage

3 medium radishes, cubed

1 mini cucumber, cubed (about ½ cup)

1 medium carrot, shredded

½ avocado, cubed

10 yellow grape tomatoes, halved

2 tablespoons pumpkin seeds

FOR THE DRESSING:

⅓ cup apple cider vinegar

2 tablespoons spicy brown mustard

½ teaspoon garlic powder

Salt and pepper to taste

1. Combine all salad ingredients in a large bowl.
2. Combine all of the dressing ingredients and mix until blended.
3. Pour the dressing over the salad.

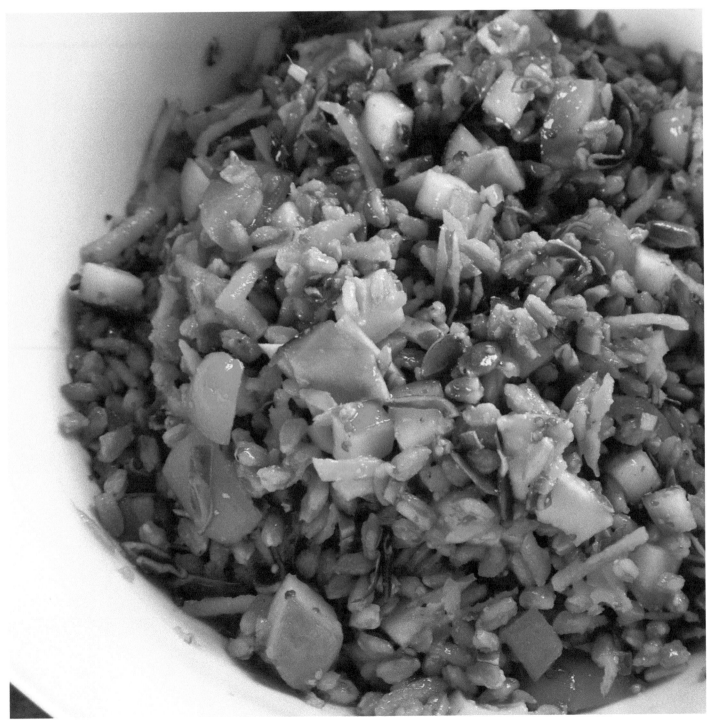

PURPLE DOG SALAD

Serves 2

*When we lived on our lavender farm
(Purple Dog Farm) we used to eat this
salad a lot!*

6 cups of greens (lettuce, spinach, baby kale, field greens, etc)

1 large beet cut into bite sized pieces

⅓ cup Betta than Feta (page 82)

¼ cup dried cranberries

2 tablespoons Candied Nuts (page 155)

½ cup cooked grain (quinoa, spelt, wheat berries, farro, etc)

4 tablespoons EPL Vinaigrette (page 94)

1. Toss all of the salad ingredients in a large bowl and serve.

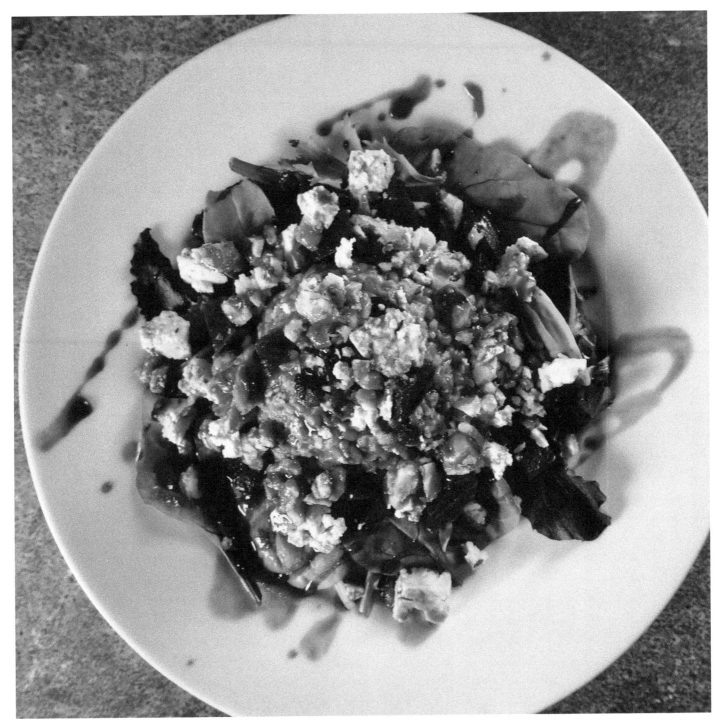

ROASTED CORN SALSA

Makes about 3 cups

2 cups frozen corn

1 small red onion, chopped

1 avocado, chopped

1 (14.5 oz.) can fire roasted tomatoes, drained

1 red pepper, chopped

3 garlic cloves, minced

4 tablespoons lime juice

salt and pepper to taste

1. In a skillet, dry sauté corn until it begins to brown. Remove from heat, set aside and let cool.

2. Place all the ingredients in a bowl and mix to combine.

3. Refrigerate until needed.

Eat Plants Love was the very first vegan cookbook I purchased and it felt like Doug and Shari were in my kitchen coaching and supporting me. After 12 months of plant-based eating it is still my go-to cookbook and I am eager to enjoy the next iteration. Remaining a plant-based vegan is so much a part of my life now. Food tastes better, I feel better and I lost 10 pounds almost effortlessly, and at my age (late sixties) that's not easy to do. The best part is I do not stress about food anymore. I no longer have to second guess or "wish I had not eaten" something because every food choice is a healthy food choice.

BJ Mann

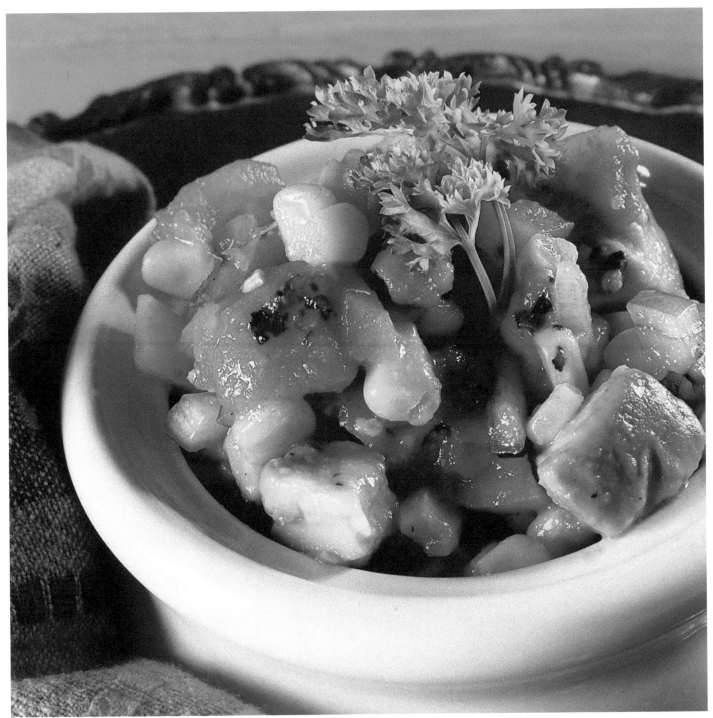

YOGURT TAHINI ROASTED CARROTS

Serves 4

4 cups carrots, sliced

¼ cup vegetable broth

3 scallions, chopped

3 cloves garlic, chopped

Salt and pepper

TAHINI DRESSING

1 cup non-dairy yogurt

¼ cup tahini

2 teaspoons lemon juice

1 teaspoon maple syrup

1. Preheat the oven to 400° F.

2. Toss carrots with broth, scallions and garlic

3. Season with salt and pepper and place on a lined baking sheet.

4. Roast until carrots are tender (about 20 minutes).

5. Drizzle with tahini sauce and serve with a whole grain such as farro, bulgur wheat or brown rice.

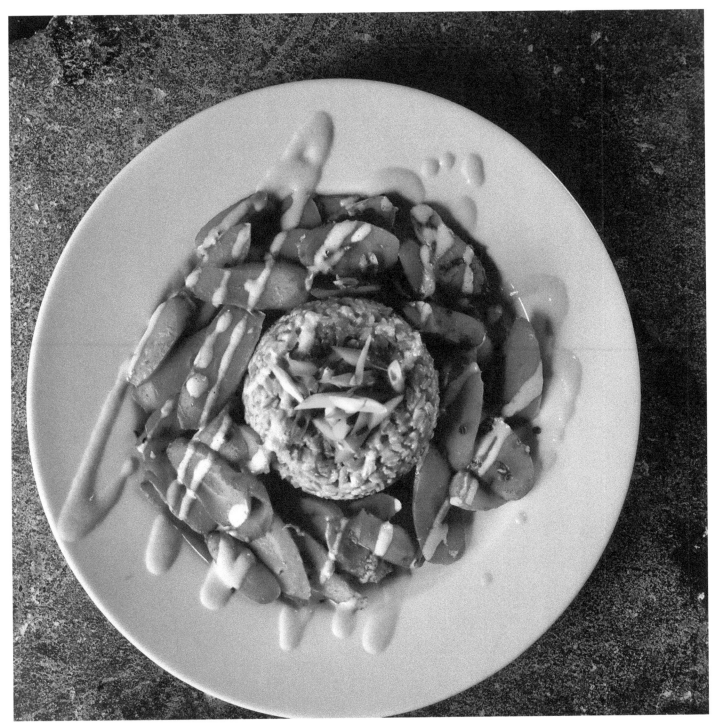

PEACH HONEYDEW SALSA

Makes about 3 cups

2 large tomatoes, diced

1 bell pepper, seeded and finely diced

1 jalapeño, seeded and finely minced

1 medium onion, finely diced

1 peach, diced

1 cup of honeydew, diced

¼ cup cilantro or parsley, chopped

2 tablespoons lime juice

1 ½ teaspoons salt, or to taste

¼ teaspoon freshly ground black pepper or to taste

1. In a medium bowl, combine all ingredients and chill until ready to use.

In 10 weeks my fasting glucose went down 23 points, from a high of 119 to 96, and my A1c went from 5.4 to 5.1. Working on continued lowering, but I'm no longer technically prediabetic!

Carol C.

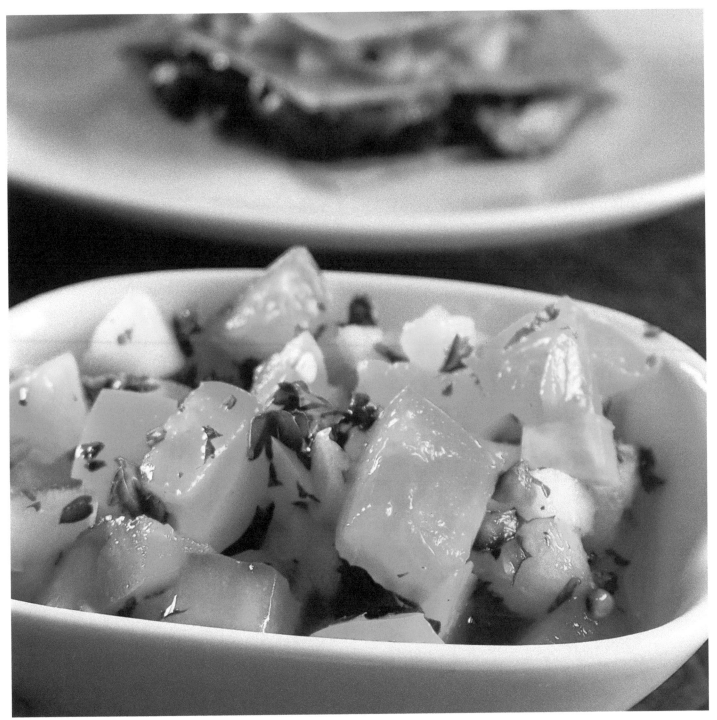

BROCCOLI CAULIFLOWER POTATO TOTS

Makes about 3 dozen

12 oz. bag frozen broccoli and cauliflower mix

¼ cup ground flax seed

¼ cup water

2 medium potatoes, peeled and diced

½ cup nutritional yeast

½ cup almond flour/meal

¼ cup potato flour

2 tablespoons dried parsley

¼ cup yellow onion, finely diced

1 teaspoon salt

1 teaspoon garlic powder

1. Preheat oven to 400°F.

2. Defrost frozen cauliflower and broccoli in the microwave for 4 minutes. Drain off any excess water.

3. Mix water and ground flax seeds together. Let it sit until thickened.

4. Place all ingredients in a food processor and pulse until uniform in texture.

5. Using a small scoop or two spoons, scoop into balls and place on a lined baking tray.

6. Bake 20-25 minutes, flip, then bake for another 20 minutes until nicely browned and crispy.

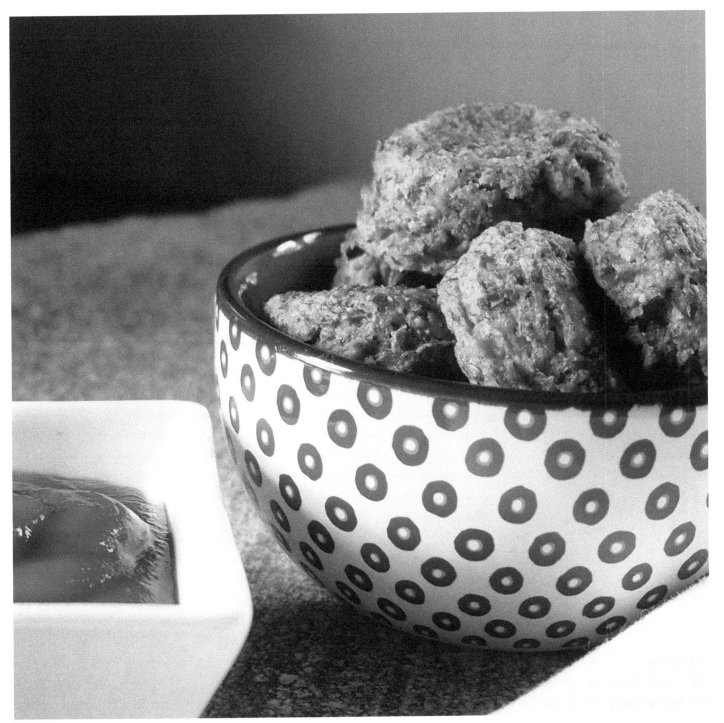

NOT "CHIKEN" STRIPS

½ bag of Butler Soy Curls™

½ cup chickpea flour

1 teaspoon poultry seasoning

1 teaspoon garlic powder

1 teaspoon onion powder

1 teaspoon smoked paprika

1 teaspoon hot sauce

¾ cup of non-dairy milk or water

Salt and pepper to taste

2 cups (or more) whole wheat panko crumbs (enough to coat all the strips)

1. Preheat oven to 400° F.

2. Place soy curls in a bowl and rehydrate with water for 8-10 minutes

3. Place all dry ingredients into a large bowl. Mix ingredients well.

4. Add hot sauce and the milk (or water) and stir until well combined. If too thick, add more liquid until the consistency of pancake batter.

5. Drain the soy curls and mix them into the batter.

6. One by one, remove the soy curls (let excess batter drip off) and toss them in panko crumbs and place on a lined cookie sheet.

7. Bake for 25-30 minutes until crispy and lightly browned.

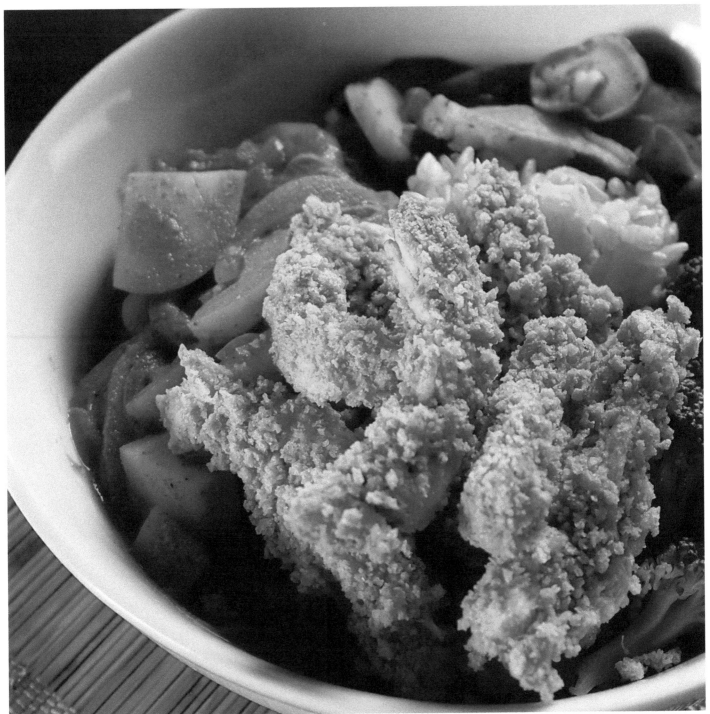

DADDY MAC SALAD

Serves 6 - 8

Submitted by Doug Pereira

Doug wanted to make a plant based garbage/trash/dumpster/compost plate using the Eat Plants Love cookbook because our group has strong ties to Rochester, NY and he was craving a garbage plate after being inspired by The Red Fern's compost plate. The Eat Plants Love cookbook had recipes for all the other ingredients (Black Bean Burgers, EPL Baked Fries, Becki's Carrot Dog Sauce) so he just wanted to figure out his own macaroni salad. Doug was kind enough to share it with us!

16 ounces whole grain pasta (elbows or bow ties work well)

1 batch of Tofu Mayonnaise (page 95)

1- 2 stalks of celery, finely chopped

1 large carrot, grated or finely chopped

Paprika to taste

Salt to taste

Black pepper to taste

1. Cook the pasta according to directions.
2. Drain the pasta and run under cold water to cool.
3. Mix all the ingredients in a large bowl.
4. Chill in the refrigerator for at least 2 hours before serving.

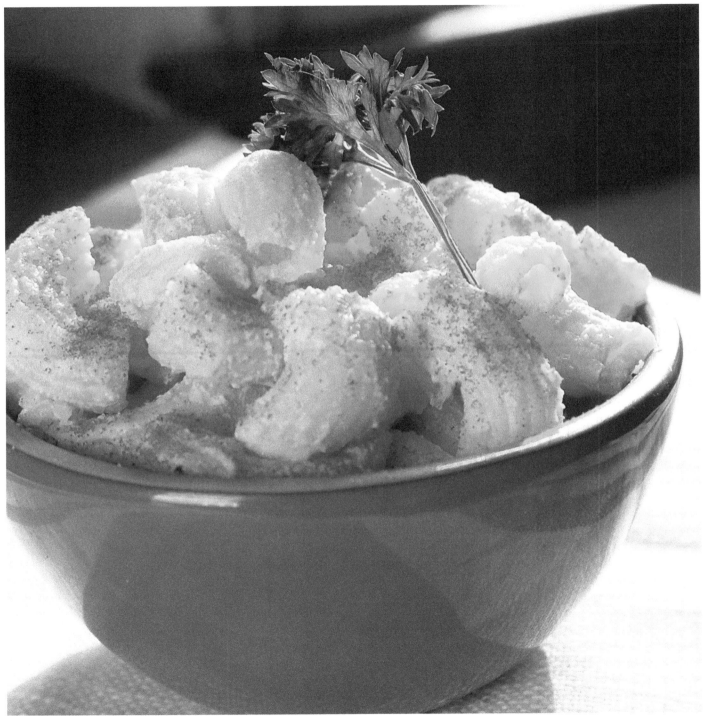

BETTA THAN FETA

1 package extra firm tofu, drained, pressed and cubed

BRINE

1 cup water

¼ cup red wine vinegar

½ teaspoon salt

2 garlic cloves, crushed

MARINADE

1 tablespoon mild miso paste

1 teaspoon dried oregano

2 tablespoons fresh lemon juice

½ teaspoon maple syrup

1. Cube tofu.

2. Combine brine ingredients and soak the tofu in the brine for 30 minutes. Drain.

3. Mix marinade ingredients. Toss tofu in marinade and refrigerate for at least an hour (or overnight).

4. Serve cubed or crumbled over a salad.

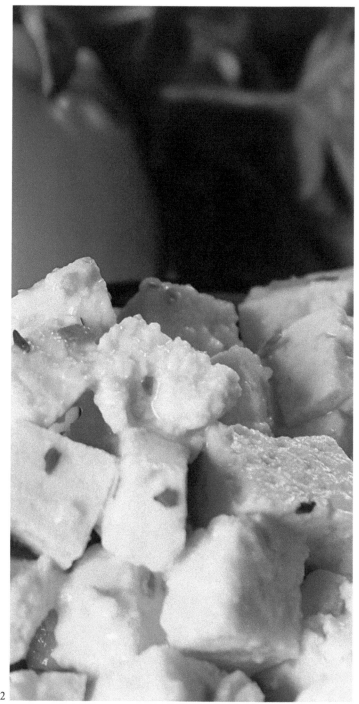

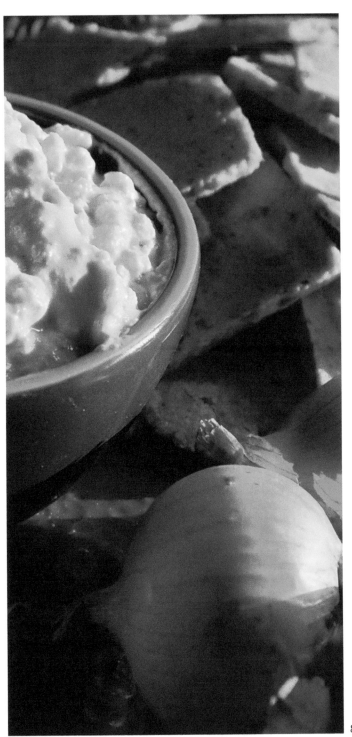

EPL ONION SOUP MIX

Yields approximately 1 cup

¼ teaspoon celery seeds

¾ cup dried minced onions

⅓ cup mushroom powder (see notes)

1 tablespoon plus 1 teaspoon onion powder

¼ teaspoon freshly ground pepper

¼ teaspoon paprika

1. Chop or grind the celery seeds to break them up a little. (You can do this with the back of a chef's knife.)

2. Place all the ingredients in a jar with a lid and shake.

NOTES

We buy dehydrated shiitake mushrooms in the Asian food section of our supermarket. We then place them in our blender and pulverize and store in a covered container until needed to add to soups and stews.

For a rich addition to soups we combine 2 tablespoons of the onion mix with 2 teaspoons of Marmite ™ (yeast spread, could also use Vegemite ™) and 2 teaspoons of soy sauce to 1/2 cup of hot water.

STUFFED MUSHROOMS

We try to include mushrooms into our diet as much as possible. This is one of our favorite ways to do that.

14-16 medium sized portobello mushrooms (1 ½ inch across)

1 small onion, minced

2 cloves of garlic, crushed

vegetable broth as needed

¼ cup of red wine or a splash of balsamic vinegar, or both

1 tablespoon vegan worcestershire sauce

1 tablespoon fresh thyme

1 tablespoon fresh oregano

½ cup whole wheat bread crumbs *

¼ cup nutritional yeast

salt and pepper

You could also use whole wheat panko crumbs, chickpea crumbs, ground oats or some other binding ingredient.

1. Preheat the oven to 400° F.

2. Pull stems from mushrooms and set aside. Place caps in a shallow baking dish, gill side facing up.

3. Chop stems into fine pieces to yield 1½ cups of chopped mushroom bits. Chop extra mushrooms if needed.

4. Sauté mushroom stems/pieces in broth with the onions and garlic until tender.

5. Add thyme, salt and pepper.

6. Add wine/vinegar and cook until wine has evaporated.

7. Take off of heat, add bread crumbs and nutritional yeast. This should form a mix that holds somewhat together when picked up on a spoon. If not, add a bit more liquid until it holds together.

8. Place a spoonful of mushroom mix on top of each cap.

9. Bake for 20-30 minutes until mushrooms are cooked through. Serve warm.

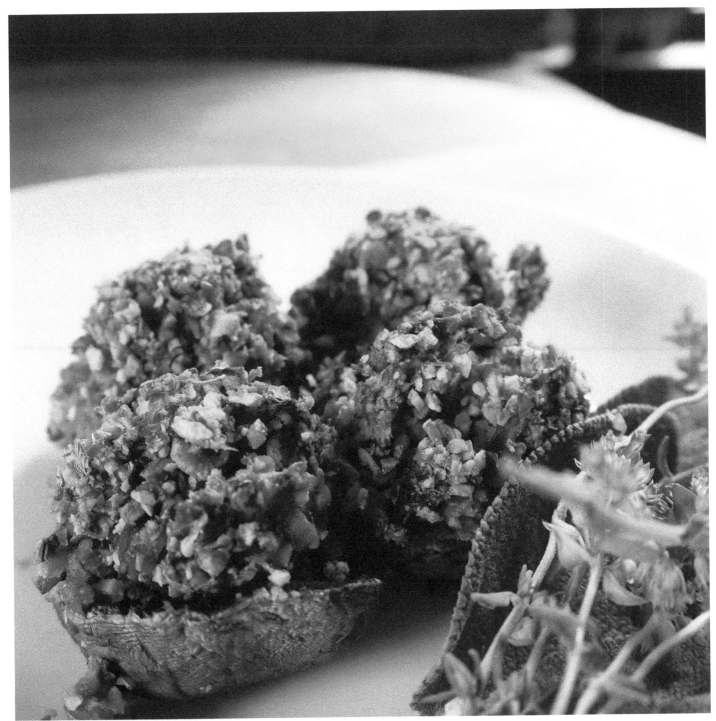

MARINATED SHIITAKE MUSHROOMS

2 cups sliced shiitake mushrooms

Marinade

¼ cup low sodium soy sauce (make sure it is low sodium otherwise it will be too salty)

⅛ cup maple syrup

⅛ cup rice vinegar

3 dashes of liquid smoke

1. Combine marinade ingredients in a bowl and add the mushrooms and toss to coat evenly. Marinate the sliced mushrooms for at least ½ hour.

2. Drain the mushrooms (reserving some of the marinade) and sauté until nicely colored. Add marinade to the pan, if needed, to prevent the mushrooms from sticking.

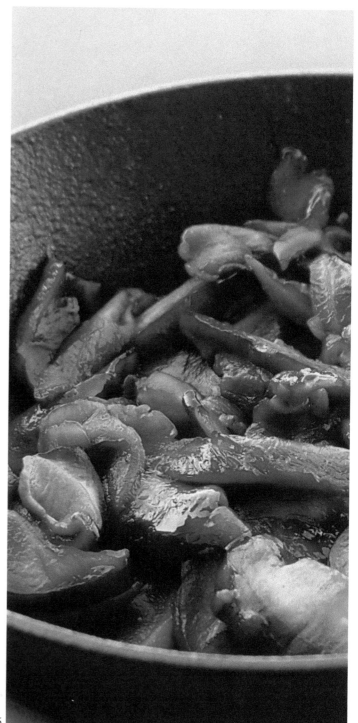

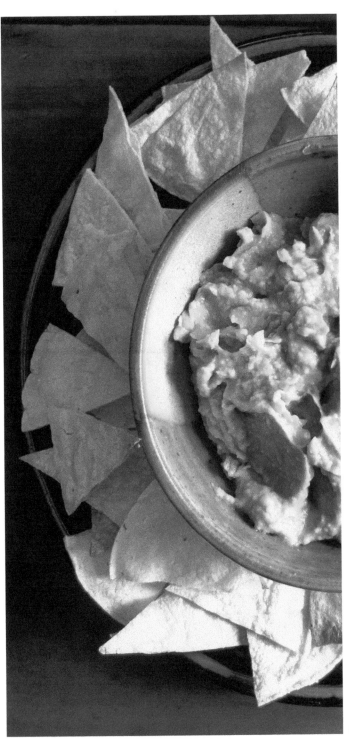

HOLY GUACAMOLE

Makes about 1 cup

1 avocado

2 tablespoons salsa

1 clove garlic, chopped

½ teaspoon onion powder

½ teaspoon garlic powder

2 teaspoons lime juice

salt and pepper to taste

hot sauce to taste

1. Cut lengthwise around the avocado.

2. Twist and separate the avocado halves. Use a knife embedded in the pit and twist to remove.

3. Scoop the avocado into a food processor. Add the rest of the ingredients and process.

4. Add salt, pepper and hot sauce to taste.

5. Serve with oil-free tortilla chips.

"No disease that can be treated by diet should be treated with any other means."

Maimonides

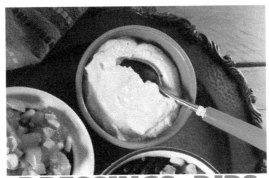

DRESSINGS, DIPS AND SAUCES

GINGER MISO DRESSING

Makes about 1 ½ cups

½ cup white miso

4 tablespoons maple syrup

½ cup rice vinegar

1 tablespoon toasted sesame seeds

2 tablespoons tahini

2 tablespoons grated fresh ginger

2 cloves garlic

1 tablespoon lemon juice

1. Blend all ingredients until smooth and refrigerate until ready to use. Shake well before serving.

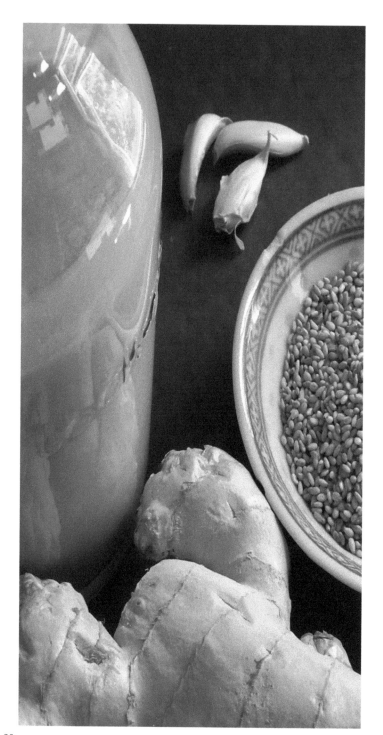

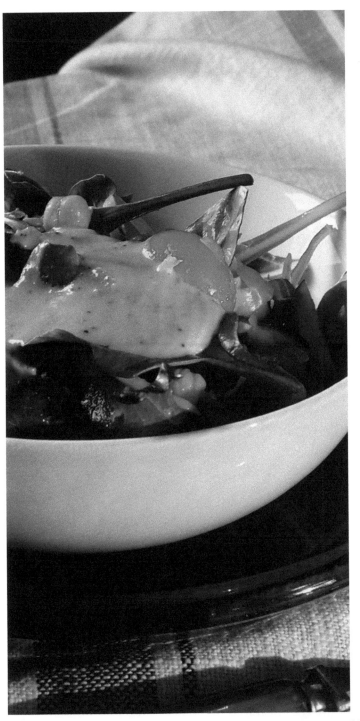

POPPY SEED DRESSING

Makes 1 cup

½ cup raw sunflower seeds, soaked for 30 minutes then drained

½ cup cider vinegar

3-4 tablespoons maple syrup

1 teaspoon Dijon mustard

½ teaspoon sweet paprika

¾ teaspoon salt

½ teaspoon onion powder

3 tablespoons water

1 - 1 ½ tablespoons poppy seeds

1. Blend everything except poppy seeds until smooth.
2. Add poppy seeds and stir to combine.

FRENCH DRESSING

Makes 1 cup

Shari loves French dressing and wanted a healthy variation. Sunflower seeds are so beneficial to our health and this is an easy way to get them into your diet. Sunflower seeds are an excellent source of vitamin E, magnesium, and selenium. These are nutrients often missing in our diets.

½ cup raw sunflower seeds, soaked

¼ cup white vinegar

¼ cup cider vinegar

4 tablespoons maple syrup

1 teaspoon vegan worcestershire sauce

1 teaspoon Dijon mustard

1 teaspoon sweet paprika

1 clove garlic

¾ teaspoon salt

½ teaspoon garlic powder

½ teaspoon onion powder

1. Blend everything in a blender until smooth.
2. Refrigerate until ready to use.

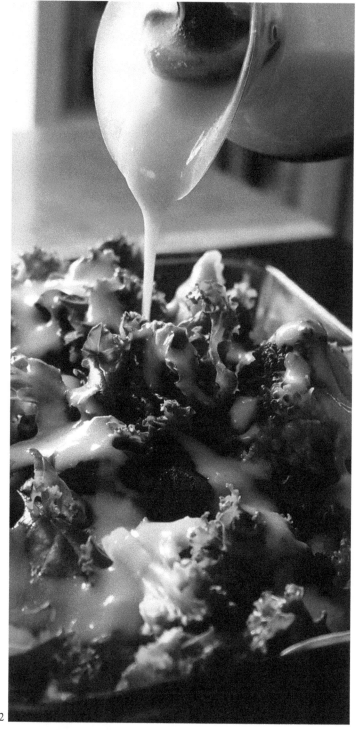

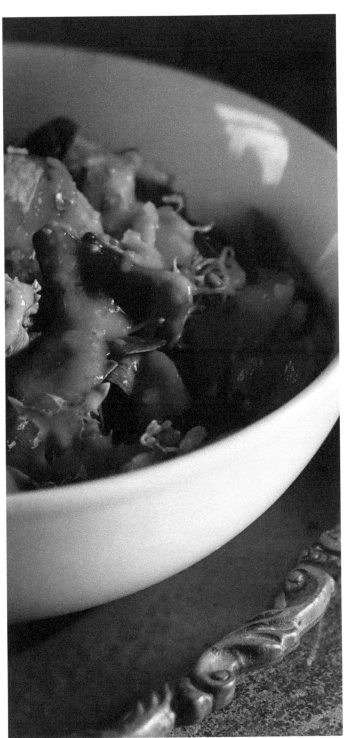

RED PEPPER VINAIGRETTE WITH MISO

Yields about 1 ¼ cups

Miso is a fermented product. Naturally fermented products are great for your gut microbiome. Miso is a good source of a number of minerals, such as copper, manganese, phosphorus, and zinc. Add this delicious dressing to your arsenal!

¼ cup white miso

¼ cup water

½ cup roasted red pepper, chopped (jarred works)

3 dates, chopped

¼ cup apple cider vinegar

1 garlic clove

½ tablespoon chopped red onion

½ tablespoon soy sauce

1 teaspoon dried basil

1 teaspoon oregano

1. Blend everything in a blender until smooth.
2. Refrigerate until ready to use.

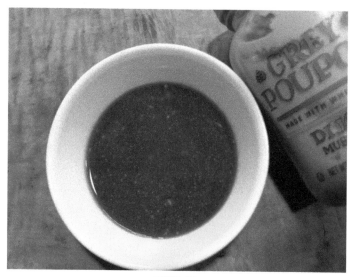

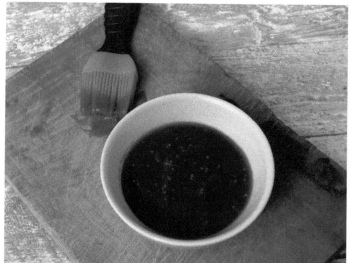

EPL VINAIGRETTE

Our go-to quick and easy dressing.

6 tablespoons balsamic or apple cider vinegar

4 tablespoons Dijon mustard

3 tablespoons maple syrup

1. Place all ingredients in jar and shake it up until combined.

OIL-FREE BBQ SAUCE

Makes 1 ½ cups

1 cup ketchup

1 tablespoon coarse ground mustard

2 tablespoons maple syrup

1 tablespoon cider vinegar

2 teaspoons vegan worcestershire sauce

1 teaspoon smoked paprika

7-8 drops liquid smoke (optional)

hot sauce to taste (optional)

¼ cup water or more

1. Place everything in a bowl (except the water) and mix well.

2. Add water, a bit at a time, until you get the consistency you desire.

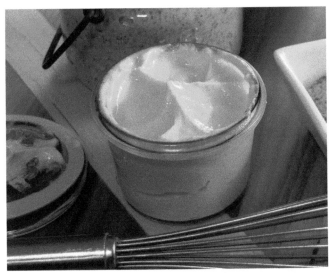

TOFU MAYONNAISE

Makes 1 cup

¼ cup raw cashews, soaked for at least 4 hours

7 oz. firm tofu, drained

4 teaspoons lemon juice

½ tablespoon rice vinegar

2 tablespoons cider vinegar

1 tablespoon Dijon mustard

1 ½ tablespoons maple syrup

½ teaspoon salt

1. Place all of the ingredients in a blender and blend until smooth. Scrape down periodically and blend some more.
2. Store in a refrigerator for up to a week.

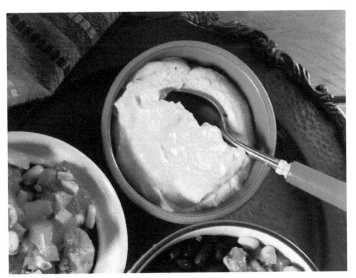

EPL SOUR CREAM

Makes about 1 ¼ cups

¾ cup raw sunflower seeds, soaked for 30 minutes then drained

½ cup plain non-dairy yogurt

4 tablespoons lemon juice

¾ tablespoon apple cider vinegar

¾ teaspoon salt

Water to thin

1. Place everything in a blender and blend until smooth and creamy. Gradually add water to thin to proper consistency.

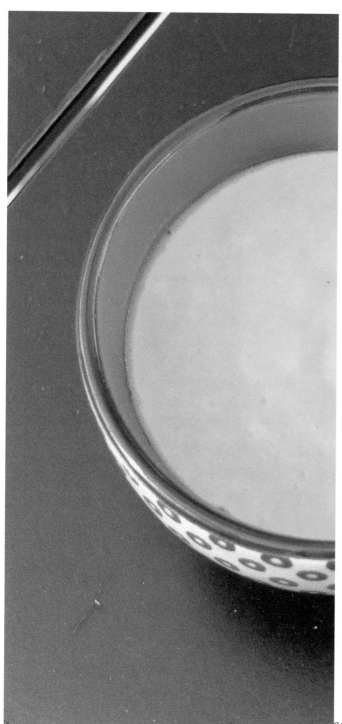

MELISSA'S CHEEZ SAUCE

Makes 3 1/2 cups

2 cups of potatoes, peeled and diced

1 cup carrots, peeled and diced

½ cup water

½ cup nutritional yeast

2 teaspoons salt (you can use less if you want)

1 tablespoon lemon juice

¼ teaspoon garlic powder

¼ teaspoon onion powder

⅛ teaspoon cayenne pepper (or more to taste)

1. Boil potatoes and carrots until soft.

2. Place all ingredients in blender or a food processor and blend them until smooth.

3. Add water to thin to desired consistency.

Thank You Melissa O'Grady!

"In the world of medicine, if I put you on a pill, I can see you every three months for the rest of your life. That's how we make money in medicine. If I put you on a plant based diet and you get better, I probably won't see you again."

Dr. James Bennie MD, Family Physician

CANNELLINI HUMMUS

Yields 1 ¾ cups

A creamy twist on traditional hummus

½ cup raw cashews, soaked

1 (15 oz.) can cannellini beans, drained and rinsed

1 clove garlic

1 teaspoon lemon juice

1 teaspoon cumin

¼ cup water

Salt and pepper to taste

1. Blend all the ingredients until smooth and creamy.

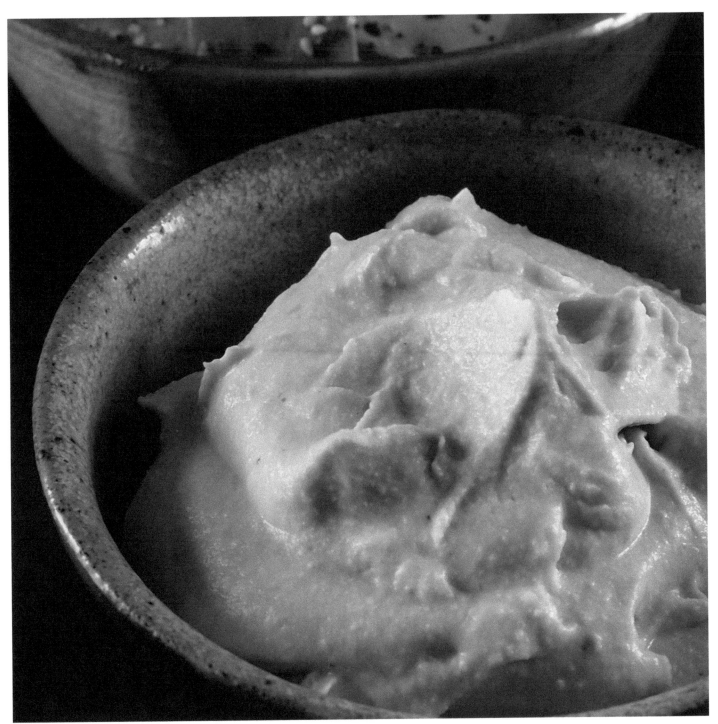

FRENCH ONION DIP

*Growing up, Mom always made onion dip using the Lipton onion
soup packet. This is our take on the classic dip.*
Makes 1 ½ cups

1 batch of EPL Sour Cream (Page 95)

½ cup of EPL Onion Soup Mix (Page 83)

¼ cup water (plus extra to thin)

1. Mix the ingredients together until well blended and let onion rehydrate for a minimum of 1 hour before serving. It can be served right away, but it tastes best if refrigerated overnight. If needed, thin with extra water as the dehydrated onion will absorb moisture from the sour cream.

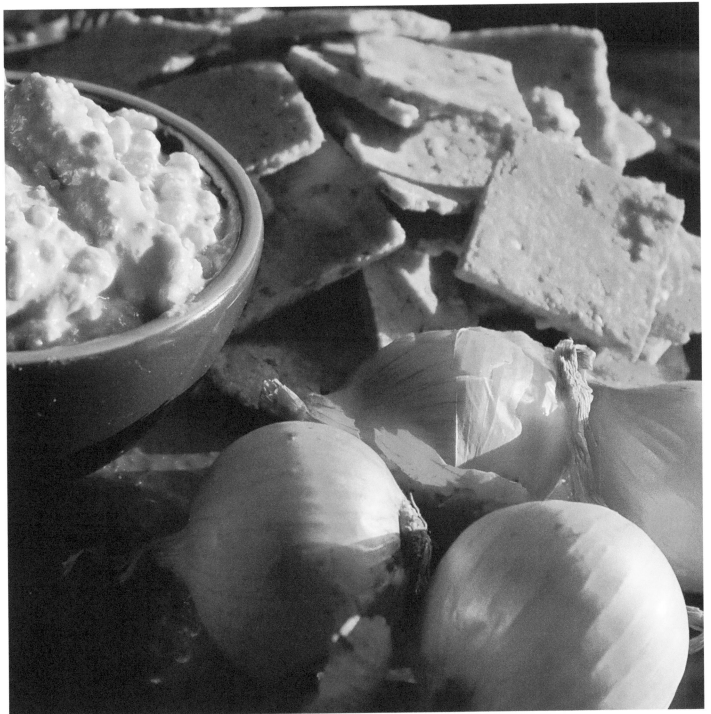

GOOD LIFE PROFILE: LYNN BROWN

"My whole food plant based journey began with my husband seeing a Joel Fuhrman segment on WXXI during a pledge drive. His 50th birthday was around the corner and he was feeling pretty lethargic. He wanted to make a change and I supported him because I was concerned about food choices he was making. My cholesterol numbers, blood pressure, and weight have always been good/normal. I do however believe that changing to a whole food plant based diet has kept me healthy after needless (in retrospect) surgery for hormonal related female issues. I say this because while I did not consume a great deal of animal products when I was younger (I did not enjoy eating more than small portions of animal flesh and did not like milk — though I did consume my fair share of cheese and ice cream) this changed around my late thirties or early forties when high protein diets became the thing and I began increasing my animal protein and dairy consumption. This is when the female health issues came to a head.

It has now been a 9 year journey. We have learned much along the way. We keep learning and improving food choices we make. We do not feel deprived as some family and friends think we do. Instead the food options seem endless. This is a good thing because we love food! I have found adapting a recipe to our plant based lifestyle more often than not results in a better version. I definitely notice a difference even if I stray for one meal (usually to be polite) that manifests in what I can only describe as a slightly heavy and hungover feeling. How I feel eating the whole food plant based way keeps me on the journey. Who knew 10 years ago that I would crave something green, even for breakfast."

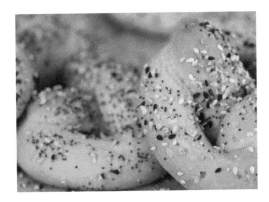

BAKED

SHARI'S OATMEAL BREAD

Makes 1 large loaf

2 cups warm water

2 tablespoons maple syrup

¼ cup unsweetened applesauce

1 pkg rapid rise yeast

3 cups whole wheat flour

½ cup oat flour

1 tsp sea salt

¼ cup raw sunflower seeds

½ cup rolled oats (plus extra for topping)

¼ cup chopped walnuts

(optional - pecans, raisins or currants ¼ cup each, Trader Joe's Everything But the Bagel Seasoning™ on top.)

Note: If it seems like there is too much dough, put some in a muffin tin. Remove from the oven 5 –8 minutes before the loaf.

Based on Kim Cambell's recipes in both her books: Plant Pure Nation and Plant Pure Kitchen.

1. In a small bowl mix water, maple syrup, applesauce and yeast. Let stand for 10 minutes.

2. In large bowl, mix the flours, salt, sunflower seeds, ½ cup oats, and the nuts (and optional nuts and dried fruit).

3. Mix the wet ingredients into the dry (for about 3 minutes- vigorously) until all incorporated. It will be sticky but you shouldn't be able to knead it.

4. Place the dough into a parchment paper-lined large loaf pan (or silicone pan) or 2 small loaf pans.. Sprinkle some oats on top. Cover and let it sit for about 1 ½ hours.

5. Note: The bread rises pretty high in a large loaf pan. I use this size to make sandwich bread. The dough will actually fill 2 small loaves. Keep an eye on the rise. When it puffs up over the top, it is ready to go into the oven. Depending on the temperature in your kitchen, it may take a little less or more time to rise.

6. Preheat the oven to 350°F. Uncover the bread and bake for about 45 - 50 minutes, covering halfway through with tented aluminum foil. It should be lightly browned on top.

7. Remove from the oven and let it cool for 20 minutes. Turn it out onto a rack and cool before slicing.

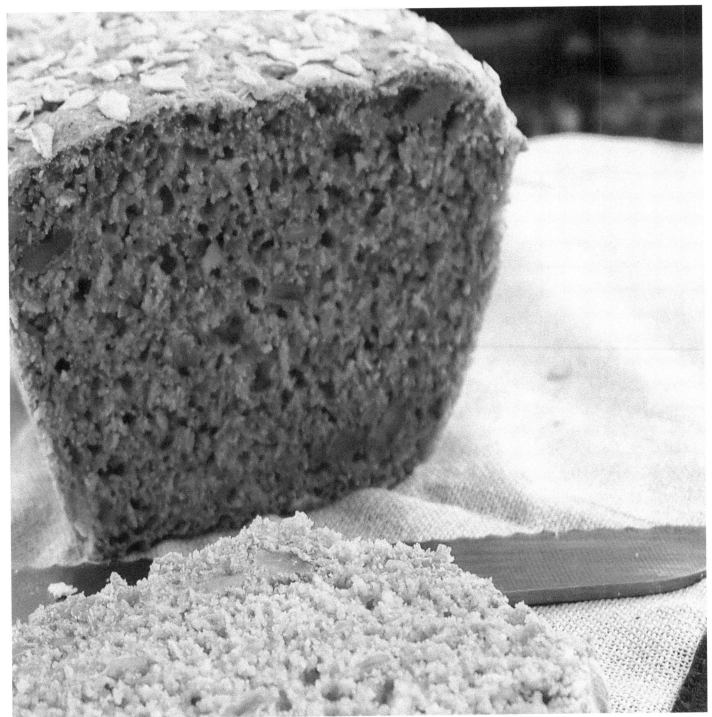

PEANUT BUTTER BREAD

The original, no-yeast peanut butter bread first circulated in a 1932 cookbook from the Five Roses Flour company. We made it all from plants and a little healthier.

Makes 1 loaf

1 ½ cups whole wheat flour

½ cup oat flour

4 teaspoons baking powder

½ teaspoon salt

1 ⅓ cups non-dairy milk

¼ cup maple syrup

½ cup peanut butter (made from just peanuts, no oil added)

½ cup non-dairy chocolate chips (optional)

1. Preheat the oven to 350° F.

2. Mix the dry ingredients in a large bowl.

3. Blend the non-dairy milk, the maple syrup and the peanut butter in a blender until smooth.

4. Fold the milk mixture into the dry ingredients. (Add the optional chocolate chips.)

5. Bake in a parchment paper lined loaf pan (or a silicone loaf pan) for 40 -45 minutes or until an inserted toothpick comes out clean.

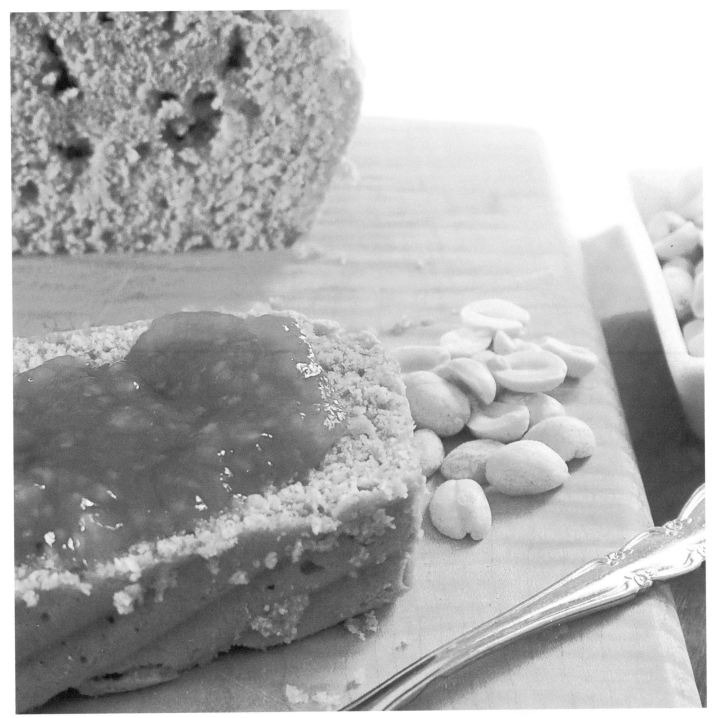

TRAILHEAD BREAD

Makes 1 loaf

Thanks to Claudia Rolnick for the original recipe.
This is our go-to bread for hiking, a canoe trip or any energy intensive adventure.

¼ cup sunflower seeds

½ cup pumpkin seeds

¾ cup sliced almonds

2 cups oats

1 cup flax seed, half of them ground

¼ cup hempseed

4 tablespoons chia seeds

⅓ cup psyllium husk powder *

¾ tablespoon sea salt

3 tablespoons maple syrup

2 ½ cups water

1. Preheat the oven to 350°F.

2. Toast sunflower seeds, pumpkin seeds and almonds for 12 minutes until lightly browned.

3. Raise the oven temperature to 400°F.

4. In a large bowl, mix the toasted seeds/nuts and all the dry ingredients together (oats through salt).

5. Add the maple syrup and water and mix until thoroughly combined with no dry spots.

6. Place in a silicone loaf pan (or in a large loaf pan lined with parchment paper).

7. Bake at 400°F for about 35 minutes.

8. Gently remove the loaf from the pan, flip over onto a lined baking sheet and bake for another 15 minutes. Let it cool completely. Keeps for a few days covered, or covered in the refrigerator for longer. Freezes well.

*Psyllium husk powder is used to retain moisture and helps prevent breads from becoming too crumbly.
Note: Feel free to substitute for, or delete, the nuts if you have an allergy. Increase the amount of the sunflower and pumpkin seeds if omitting the almonds.
To make these into muffins, use a silicone or lined muffin pan and bake for 30 minutes then remove the muffins from the pan and bake for another 10 minutes.

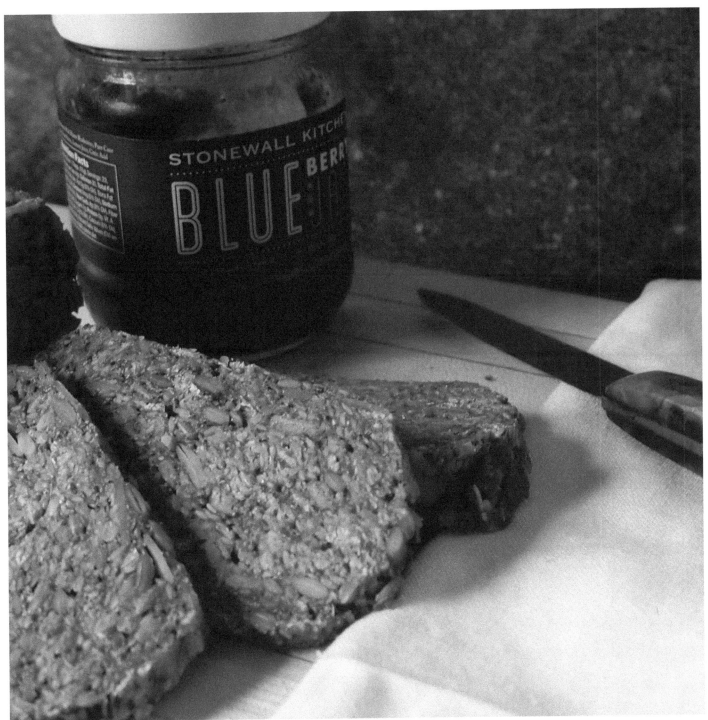

SAVORY CORN MUFFINS

Makes 10-12 muffins

1 small onion, finely chopped

½ red pepper, finely chopped

1 cup mushrooms, sliced then chopped

salt (about 1 teaspoon goes into the dry mix, a little extra goes into the veggie sauté, to taste)

pepper to taste

¾ cup frozen corn

2 large handfuls baby spinach

1 cup corn flour (if you can find it, we prefer roasted corn flour for more flavor)

1 cup whole wheat flour

½ cup nutritional yeast

1 tablespoon baking powder

½ teaspoon turmeric

½ teaspoon garlic powder

½ teaspoon dried thyme (or 1 tablespoon fresh)

½ teaspoon Aleppo chili powder (or your favorite chili powder)

¼ cup applesauce

1 cup non-dairy milk

1. Preheat the oven to 400°F.

2. Sauté onion, pepper and mushrooms until soft and starting to brown.

3. Add a little salt and pepper to taste.

4. Put the corn in a medium bowl.

5. Add the sautéed vegetables to the frozen corn. (This cools off the veggies before adding to the muffin mix and helps to thaw corn)

6. Steam the spinach. When cooled, squeeze out the excess moisture and finely chop.

7. In a separate bowl, add all the dry ingredients and seasonings and 1 teaspoon of salt. Stir well.

8. Add the applesauce and milk to the dry ingredients and stir until just incorporated.

9. Add the vegetable/spinach mixture to the batter and stir until combined.

10. Portion out into a silicone muffin pan and bake at 400°F for 20 minutes.

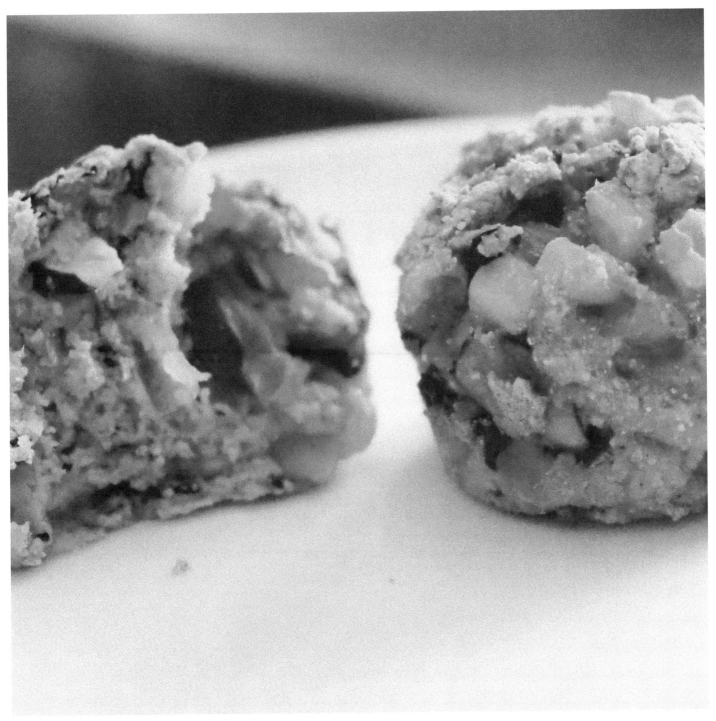

OAT ROLLS

Makes 1 dozen

1 ½ cups water (room temperature)

1 cup non-dairy milk (room temperature)

½ cup maple syrup

1 package of yeast

3 cups whole wheat bread flour

1 cup oat flour

½ cup potato flour

2 ½ teaspoons salt

Toppings: rolled oats, wheat bran, sunflower seeds, sesame seeds, poppy seeds or Trader Joe's Everything But the Bagel Seasoning™.

1. In a large bowl mix the water, milk, maple syrup and yeast together. Let it stand for 5 minutes.

2. Add 2 cups of the wheat flour and mix until uniform. Let it stand for 20 minutes.

3. Add the rest of the flours and mix until fully incorporated.

4. Sprinkle the salt on top of the dough and work it into the dough. Keep kneading the dough until smooth and elastic (about 10 minutes). Place in a bowl, cover and let rise until double in size. Depending on the warmth of the kitchen and the warmth of the dough, this could take 30 minutes up to over an hour.

5. Remove the dough from the bowl and shape into one big long round loaf. Let rest for 10 minutes.

6. Cut the dough into 12 portions.

7. Using your hands, roll the dough into balls. This is done by palming the dough in one hand and rolling the ball on the counter with gentle pressure from your cupped hand, moving in a circular motion.

8. Gently press a topping of your choice into the dough (or leave plain). Place on a lined baking sheet.

9. Let rise covered for 30-45 minutes until almost double the size.

10. Bake at 400°F for 5 minutes and reduce the heat to 350° F for remaining minutes (about 20 minutes).

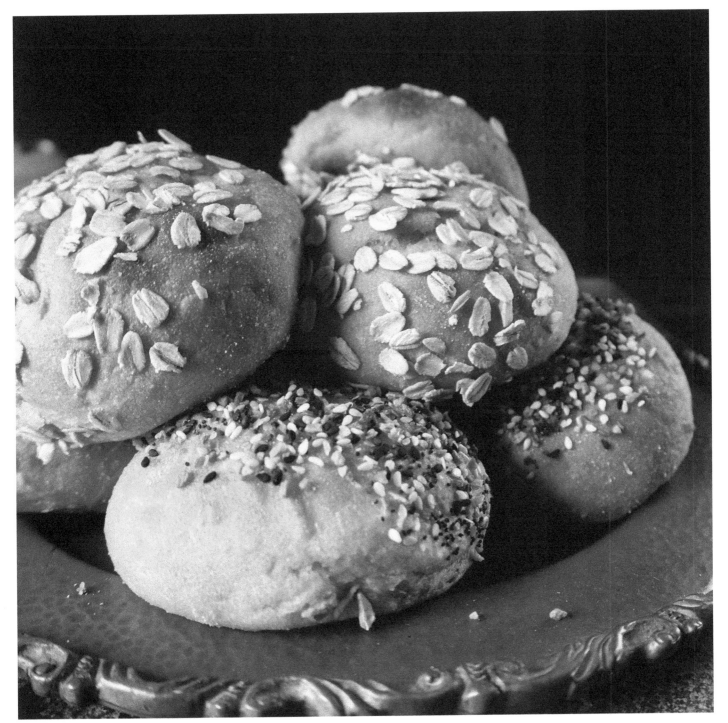

WHOLE WHEAT SOFT PRETZELS

Makes 8 pretzels

1 package active dry yeast

Liquid from one can of chickpeas (aquafaba)

½ cup water

1 tablespoon maple syrup

3 cups whole wheat flour

2 tablespoons non-diastatic malt powder* (optional)

BATH

10 cups warm water

⅔ cup baking soda

Flake salt or pretzel salt for topping (We also like Trader Joe's Everything But the Bagel Seasoning™)

Non-diastatic malt powder is a secret ingredient bakers use to add color and sweetness. It is made from roasted barley. This is an optional ingredient. Barley malt syrup can also be used in place of the powder.

1. Combine yeast, aquafaba, water and maple syrup in a stand mixer, and mix with the paddle for one minute until somewhat combined (or just mix by hand with a wooden spoon).

2. Add the flour, malt and mix with the paddle attachment until just combined. Change to the dough hook and lower speed (#2 on a KitchenAid™) and knead for 5 minutes (10 minutes by hand). The dough should be stiff, and pull away from the side of the bowl easily. Cover the dough and let it rise at room temperature for 1 hour.

3. Preheat the oven to 450° F.

4. Remove the dough from the bowl and place onto a clean countertop. Divide the dough into 8 pieces (cut it with a knife).

5. In a large pot, combine the water and baking soda and bring to a boil.

6. Roll each of the eight pieces into a long rope, about 20 inches long, and shape each one into a pretzel.

7. Dip each pretzel into the soda bath for 30 seconds and then place on a lined baking sheet. Sprinkle with coarse sea salt, pretzel salt or dip into Trader Joe's Everything But the Bagel Seasoning™.

8. Bake for 8-10 minutes until the pretzels are golden brown. We like to serve them with mustard. Yum!

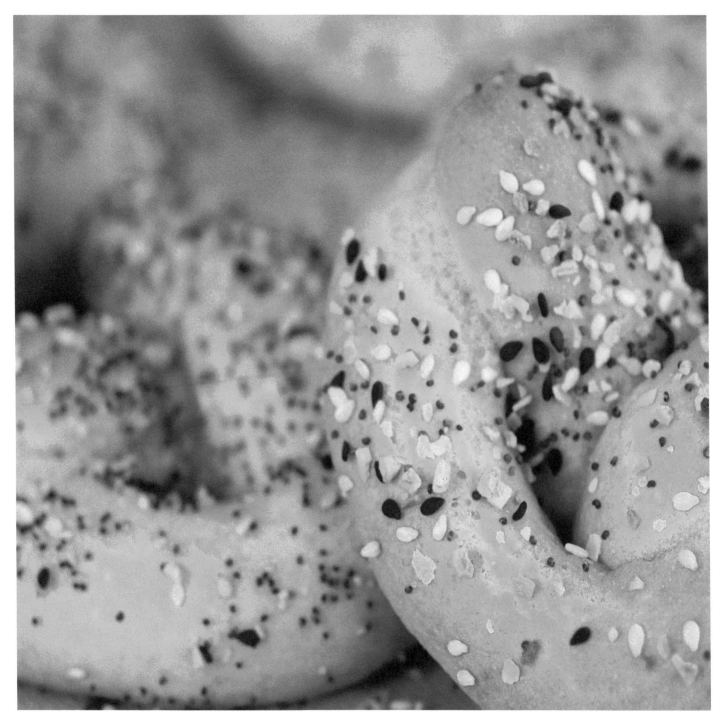

GOOD LIFE PROFILE: BARBARA KAPLAN

"I believe in this like it's a religion. I know this is more about health than weight loss but I have to say, I have been vegan for about 12 years, and slowly but surely, the scale was creeping upwards. I have struggled with weight and thyroid problems all my life, and I hadn't become vegan to lose weight--it was for the animals--but I couldn't believe how much weight I was putting on. I couldn't figure it out and was really getting depressed over this, and it's not like I think I'm 18 anymore and should be marching around in a bikini or anything. But fat = unhealthy, and too much fat = you're courting disease. I've got a mother with cardiac disease who has 7 stents and an artifical valve. My doctor, also a vegan, sent me to a WFPB-no oil workshop, and I thought, "This'll never work. I'll be the best student in the class, I won't lose an ounce, and she'll have to give me diet pills." Which is what I wanted. Four months later, I have lost 23.5 pounds, and I wasn't trying. My doc and I have laughed together over my "secret plan" to get diet pills that failed. I have thrown out every drop of oil in my house, and I'll never go back to eating and cooking the way I was. My husband weighs less than he did in college -- we've been married 30 years to give you an idea of how old we are. I've never been more satisfied in my life, and we're just starting to have grandchildren, so we need to live a LONG time!"

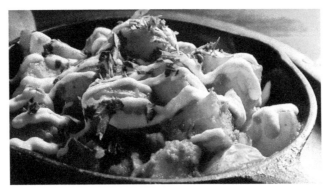

MAIN DISH IDEAS

"CHIKEN" AND DUMPLINGS

Serves 6

SOUP

1 cup yellow onion, diced

1 cup carrots, sliced

1 stalk celery, diced

3 cloves garlic cloves, minced

6 cups low sodium vegetable broth

½ cup non-dairy milk

1 teaspoon dried thyme

1 bay leaf

1 ½ cups frozen peas

5 tablespoons nutritional yeast

½ package Butler Soy Curls™ (4 oz.)

6 tablespoons whole wheat flour

6 cups low sodium vegetable broth

4 tablespoons fresh parsley, minced

Salt and pepper to taste

DUMPLINGS

2 cups whole wheat flour

1 tablespoon baking powder

1 teaspoon Italian seasoning

1 teaspoon onion powder

1 teaspoon salt

½ teaspoon pepper

1 ⅓ cups non-dairy milk

1. In a 6-quart Dutch oven, sauté onion, carrots and celery and cook until onions are just tender (about 5 minutes).

2. Add the garlic and stir until fragrant.

3. Reduce the heat to medium-low. Add the vegetable broth, non-dairy milk, thyme, and bay leaf and bring to a simmer.

4. Once the soup is at a simmer, add the frozen peas, nutritional yeast and soy curls, cover, and cook for 15 minutes.

5. Remove the bay leaf.

6. Mix the flour with 7 + tablespoons of water (this is called a roux. Add enough water to make it like a thick liquid).

7. Add the roux to the pot, stirring constantly for 2 minutes to prevent lumps from forming.

8. Make the dumplings - In a large bowl, combine the flour, baking powder, Italian seasoning, onion powder, salt, pepper, and non-dairy milk. Stir until the mixture comes together into a single mass of dough (add extra flour if needed to make it come together).

9. Using a large spoon or small scoop, form the dough into small round balls about 1 inch in diameter (the dough should yield 14-16 dumplings). Drop the dough balls in the simmering soup. You want the soup to cover the dumpling so drop them from about 6 inches above the pot. Add the parsley, and cover.

10. Let the soup simmer for 15 minutes, or until the dumplings are cooked through.

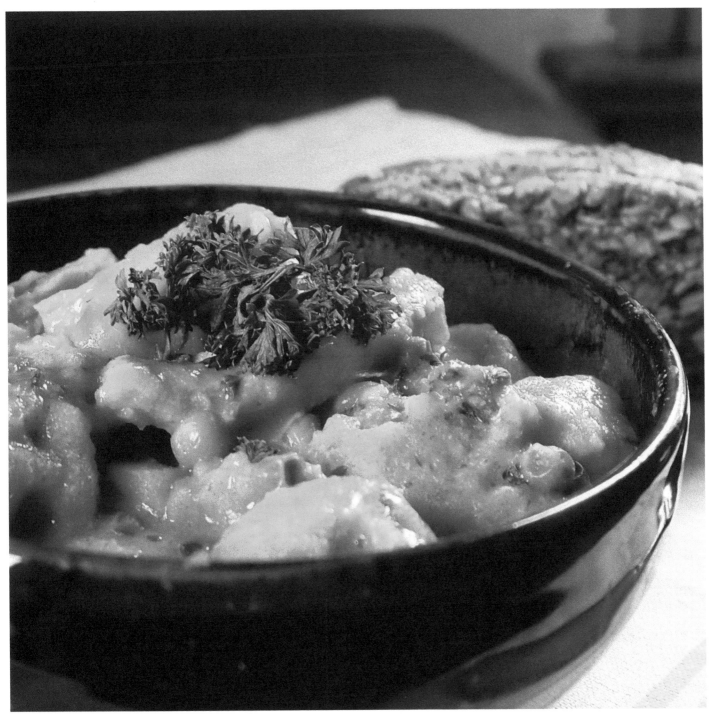

ARTICHOKE AND ROASTED RED PEPPER PASTA

Serves 4

12 ounces of whole grain pasta (bow ties or spaghetti are great)

Water, vegetable broth, vermouth or white wine for sautéing

4 cloves garlic, chopped

1 small onion, sliced into thin strips

1 cup jarred roasted red pepper (about 1 whole pepper)

¾ cup sun-dried tomatoes (rehydrated to equal 1 cup and then drained)

1 can artichokes (in water) drained and coarsely chopped

2 tablespoons Italian Seasoning

¼ - ½ teaspoon red pepper flakes

½ cup low sodium vegetable broth

3 large handfuls baby spinach

Salt and pepper to taste

Balsamic reduction

Nutritional yeast (optional)

1. Prepare pasta according to package directions. Drain and rinse with cold water. Set aside.

2. Heat a large pan (or wok) and add garlic and onions, adding some liquid to sauté for 2 minutes.

3. Add roasted red pepper, sun-dried tomatoes and artichokes and seasonings. Sauté for another 3 minutes, adding liquid if sticking.

4. Add the ½ cup vegetable broth, spinach and pasta and stir until combined. Salt and pepper to taste.

5. Drizzle balsamic reduction on top, add optional nutritional yeast and serve.

Note: We like to add mushrooms to the onions and garlic. We add mushrooms whenever possible!

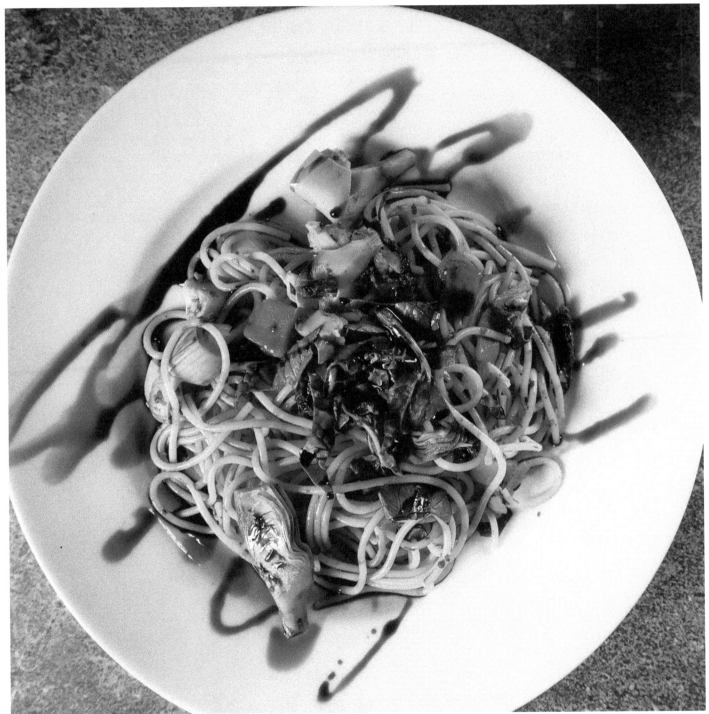

SWEET POTATO GNOCCHI

Makes about 5 dozen

1 cup cooked sweet potato, mashed

1 cup firm tofu, drained

½ cup nutritional yeast

1 ½ teaspoons salt

¾ cup whole wheat bread flour

brown rice flour for dusting

1. Mix everything except the flours until smooth and somewhat uniform.

2. Add the whole wheat bread flour and mix until it holds together.

3. Lightly dust your work surface with a little brown rice flour. Take a handful of dough and roll and shape it into a long cylinder about 1 inch in diameter.

4. Cut one inch pieces from the cylinder. Place them on a floured (brown rice) tray.

5. Boil for 2-4 minutes in lightly salted water until gnocchi floats to the top. Serve with your favorite sauce.

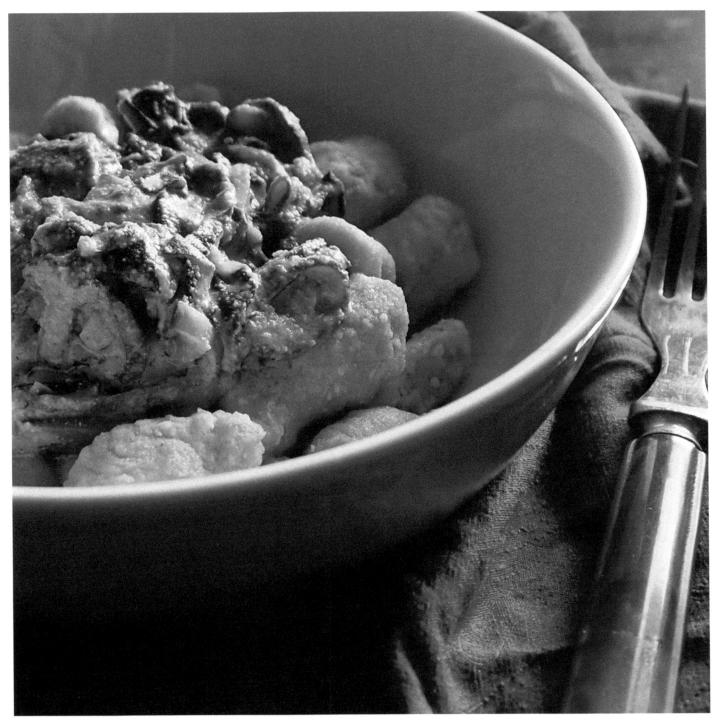

SHIITAKE MUSHROOM STACK

Serves 4

Spicy Corn Tortillas cut into 3 X 3 squares, 3 per person (Page 125)

1 (15 oz.) can black beans, drained and rinsed *

Marinated Shiitake Mushrooms (Page 86)

Holy Guacamole (Page 87)

Peach Honeydew Salsa (Page 74)

Parsley or cilantro, chopped

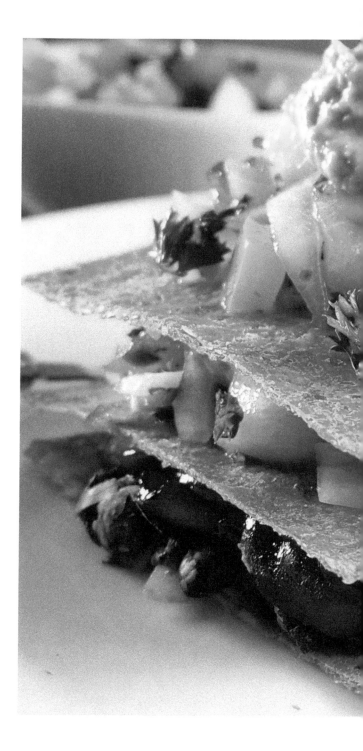

I. Place a tortilla square on the plate and top with a layer of blackbeans and Marinated Shiitake Mushrooms, add another layer of tortilla then add some Holy Guacamole and some Peach Melon Salsa and then place the other square and top with more salsa and guacamole. Top with some chopped parsley or cilantro and serve.

Note: The black beans can be added to the stack plain, or you can sauté them with a little garlic and chopped onion for added flavor.

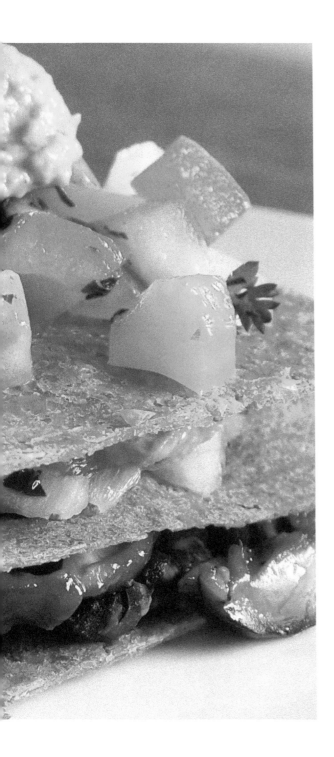

SPICY CORN TORTILLAS

*Serves 4 (plus leftover scraps) The cut pieces can
be frozen or stored in a container for up to a week.*

3 cups fresh corn kernels or frozen corn, thawed but not
cooked
1 ½ cups yellow or red bell pepper
¾ cup ground flaxseed
2-3 tablespoons lime juice
1 teaspoon ground chili powder
1 tablespoon smoked paprika
2 teaspoons ground cumin
½ teaspoon garlic powder
½ teaspoon onion powder
1 ½ teaspoons salt

1. In a food processor, process the corn and bell
pepper. Add ground flaxseed, lime juice, chili powder,
paprika, cumin and salt. Process until almost smooth,
but you want a little texture to the mixture.

2. Preheat the oven to 175° F (Keep Warm setting).

3. Spread the batter split between two sheet pans lined
with parchment paper or a silicone sheet. Spread the
batter until it is between ⅛ - ¼ inch thick. An offset
spatula works wonders here.

4. Bake for 90 minutes (or more) and then gently peel
and flip over onto another lined sheet pan and bake for
another 20-30 minutes. At this point they should be
leathery and still be able to bend. Cut into the shapes
you like. We cut them into 3 x3 inch squares for the
Shiitake Mushroom Stack or thin strips for salads.

BBQ SLIDERS

Serves 4

½ package Butler Soy Curls™

Oil Free BBQ sauce (page 94) or store bought oil-free barbecue sauce like Bone Suckin Sauce™

Salt and pepper, to taste

Batch of Sweet Slaw (page 62)

4 whole grain rolls or Oat Rolls (page 112)

1. Preheat oven to 375°.

2. Rehydrate the soy curls in water for 10 minutes.

3. Drain the soy curls and place them on a lined baking sheet. Season with salt and pepper. Bake for 25 minutes or until slightly crispy.

4. While the soy curls are baking, make the Sweet Slaw.

5. Once soy curls are baked, toss them in the barbecue sauce, build the sandwich and enjoy.

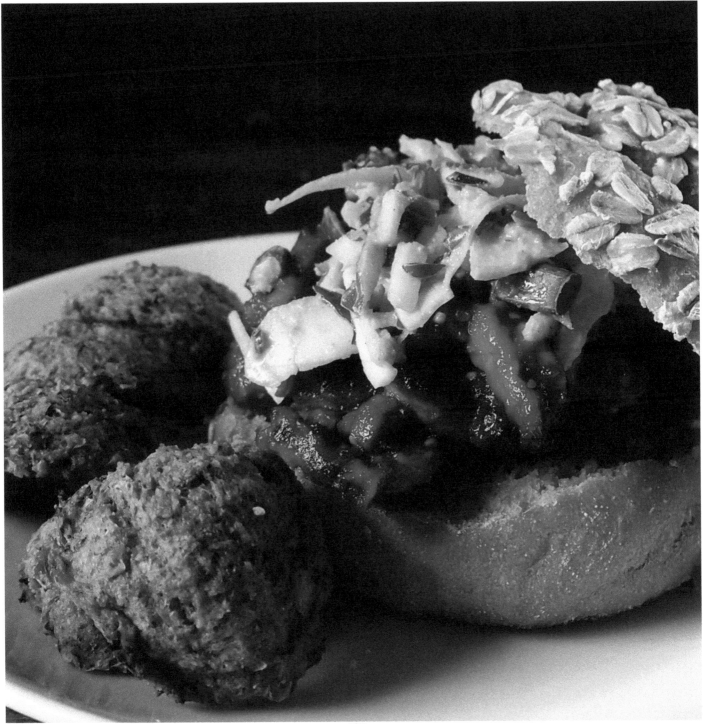

BUTLER CHEEZY BOMBER

Serves 4

1 pkg of Butler Soy Curls™

1 red pepper, cut into strips

1 onion, sliced

8 baby bella mushrooms, sliced

1 batch of Melissa's Cheez Sauce (page 96)

8 slices sourdough bread

MARINADE FOR BUTLER SOY CURLS™

½ teaspoon black pepper

1 teaspoon garlic powder

1 teaspoon onion powder

1 teaspoon ground coriander

2 teaspoon ground cumin

1 tablespoon Marmite™

2 tablespoons low sodium soy sauce

½ teaspoon chili powder

1 tablespoon hoisin sauce

1 teaspoon vegan worcestershire sauce

6 tablespoons water

1. Preheat oven to 350°F.

2. Soak the soy curls in water to rehydrate for 6-8 minutes

3. Combine the ingredients for the marinade in a medium bowl.

4. Drain the soy curls, place in the bowl with the marinade and marinate for 10 minutes.

5. Place the soy curls on silicone (or parchment paper) lined pan and bake for 20-30 minutes until crispy. (For extra spice, salt and add extra pepper before putting in the oven.)

6. While the soy curls are baking, sauté the red peppers, onions and mushrooms and set aside.

7. Make the cheeze sauce.

8. Toast your bread.

9. Top with soy curls.

10. Top with Melissa's Cheez Sauce.

11. Add the pepper, onion, mushroom mixture to the top, cover with another slice of toasted bread, slice and enjoy! Serve with greens or a green salad.

You can also use a panini maker to assemble and grill the sandwich.

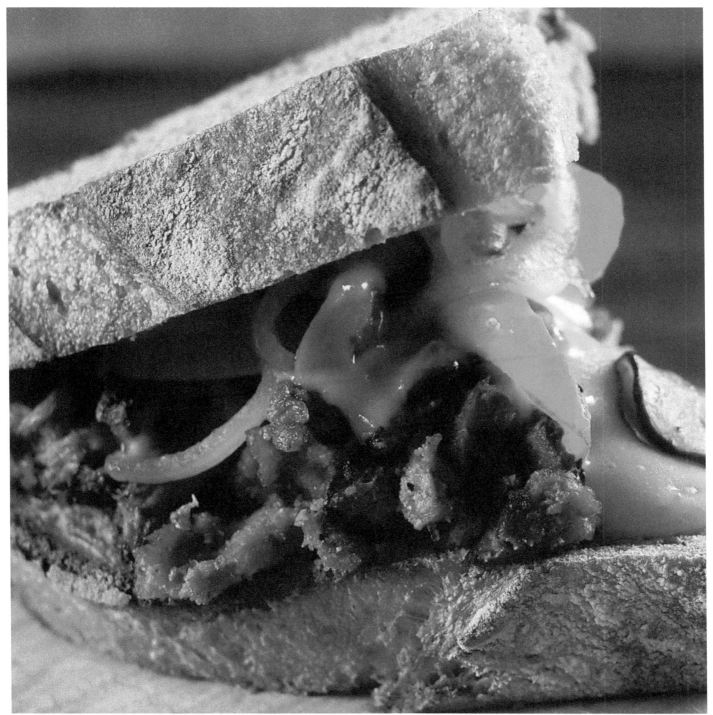

QUICK QUINOA BOWL

This recipe was submitted by Gretchen Meier–Dietrich from Gardiner, NY.

Gretchen says that she loved the quinoa bowl from Panera Bread and wanted to create something similar, but healthier, so she started making her own quinoa bowl.

Cooked quinoa - any type you like

Chopped greens (kale, spinach, lettuce)

Black beans

Cherry tomatoes

Corn or Roasted Corn Salsa (page 70)

Shallots

Chopped cilantro or parsley

Plain, unsweetened non-dairy yogurt or

EPL Sour Cream (page 95)

Salsa verde or regular salsa

1. Cook the quinoa as directed. Once done, you can allow it to cool or serve warm.

2. In a shallow bowl, place greens and 1 ½ cups of quinoa. Around the bowl place 2 tablespoons each of black beans, cherry tomatoes, and corn.

3. Dice up a ¼ of a shallot and sprinkle on top. Add chopped cilantro to taste. Top with non-dairy yogurt or sour cream, and salsa.

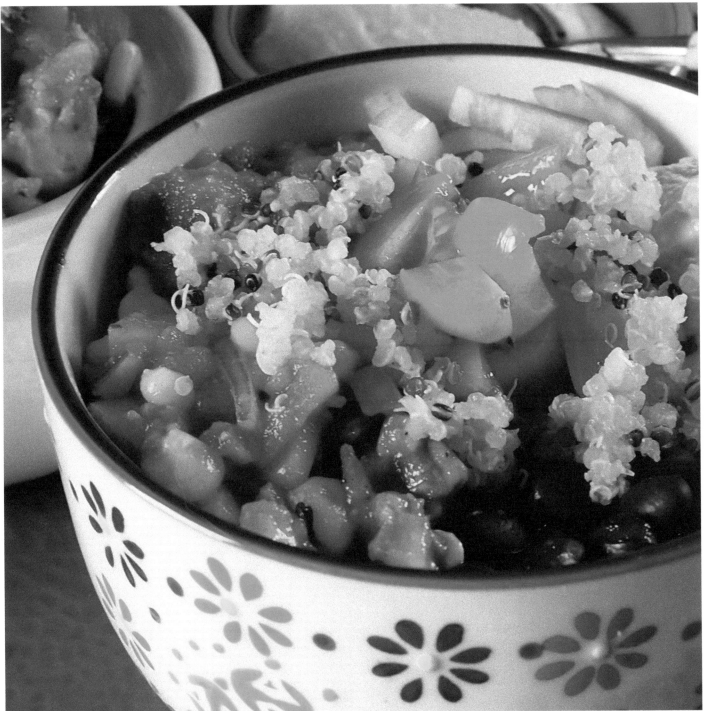

KATSU CURRY BOWL

Serves 4

Curry has a powerhouse of health benefits. This mixture of spices, besides being delicious, helps to fight inflammation and helps with cholesterol and blood flow. Curry blends vary from maker to maker, so just because you might not like one brand doesn't mean you may not like others. One of our favorite yellow curries is Maharajah curry powder from Penzey's Spices.

1 head of broccoli, chopped and steamed

2 cups shiitake mushrooms, sliced

2 cloves garlic, minced

4 cups cooked brown rice

One batch of Yellow Vegetable Curry (Page 134)

One batch of Soy Curl Katsu (Page 135)

1. Steam the broccoli for 5 minutes.

2. Sauté the mushrooms and the garlic for about 5 minutes.

3. Place ½ - 1 cup of brown rice in a bowl. Add some broccoli, some sautéed mushrooms, some Vegetable Curry and top with some Soy Curl Katsu. Serve!

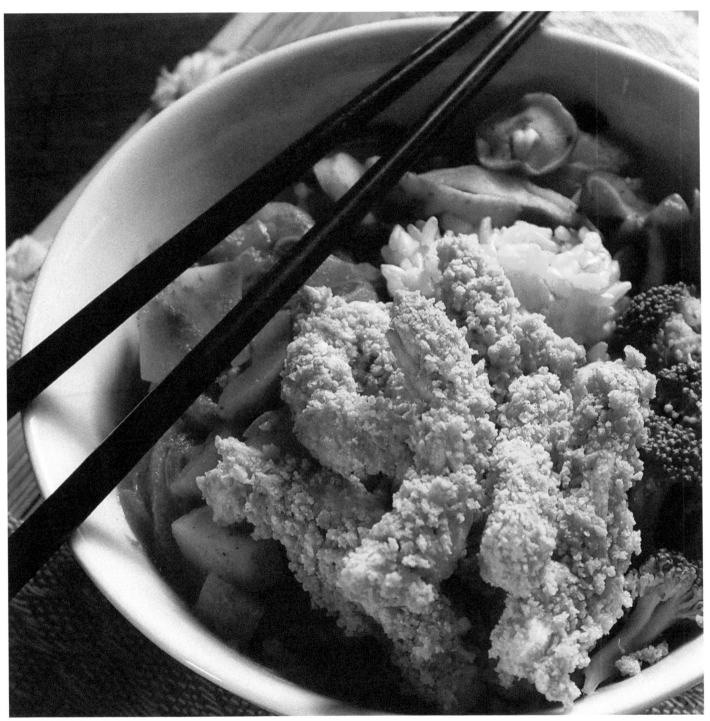

YELLOW VEGETABLE CURRY

Serves 4

1 can of unsweetened lite coconut milk (divided)

1 tablespoon yellow curry powder

1 tablespoon garam masala

3 cloves garlic, minced

¼ teaspoon cayenne pepper (optional)

1 medium onion, thinly sliced

3 tablespoons coconut aminos

2 cups vegetable broth

1 red pepper, sliced

2 carrots, sliced

1 large potato, cubed

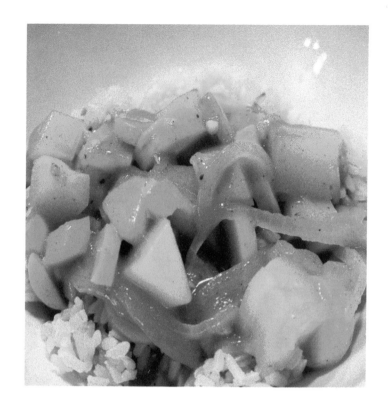

1. In a deep sauté pan, place ¼ cup coconut milk, curry powder, garam masala, garlic and optional cayenne pepper. Cook over medium heat, stirring the mixture until the kitchen fills with the aroma of the spices.

2. Add sliced onion and cook until softened. If the mixture gets too dry, add a tablespoon of water/broth as needed.

3. Add the coconut aminos and stir.

4. Add the vegetable broth and the red pepper, carrots and potato and stir to combine. Bring to a simmer. Cover and lower the heat and cook until the potatoes and carrots are tender. About 25-30 minutes.

5. Once the carrot and potatoes are tender, pour in the rest of the coconut milk and bring back to a simmer.

6. In a small bowl, mix the cornstarch and water into a slurry. Add to the curry and stir until thickened.

7. Salt and pepper to taste. Serve over rice and/or a bed of baby spinach.

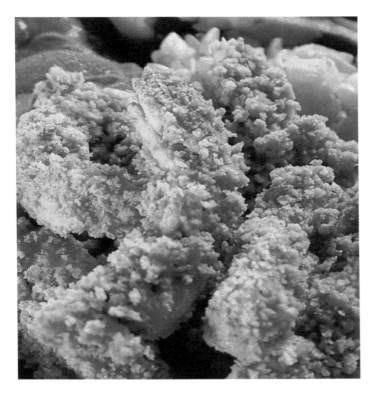

SOY CURL KATSU

½ bag Butler Soy Curls™

Batter

1 cup chickpea (garbanzo) flour

1 teaspoon garlic powder

1 teaspoon onion powder

1 teaspoon salt

1 teaspoon turmeric

½ teaspoon black pepper

1 cup water

2 cups whole wheat panko crumbs

1. Preheat the oven to 375° F.

2. Rehydrate soy curls in a bowl with water.

3. In a medium size bowl, add all the batter ingredients except the water.

4. Stir the dry ingredients and gradually add the water until the mixture coats a spoon nicely without being too runny. If runny, add more flour. If too thick, add more water. It should have the consistency of pancake batter.

5. Once the soy curls are softened, drain them and place them in the batter and stir to coat all the curls.

6. In a separate bowl or a large ziplock bag, place the panko crumbs.

7. Take the soy curls out of the batter (let the excess batter drip off). Place the soy curls into the panko crumbs and stir to coat, or if using the ziplock bag, seal and shake until all the pieces are coated.

8. Place the soy curls onto a parchment paper/ silicone lined baking sheet.

9. Bake the soy curls for 20 minutes, turn and bake for another 20 minutes until starting to get crispy.

GREEN COCONUT CURRY VEGETABLES

Serves 4

"A colleague/friend of mine told me that I should try Thai Brand Green Curry Paste. I needed a quick recipe for dinner and I love curry. I used ingredients that I had at home since my colleague/friend gifted me a bottle of the curry paste. Glad I gave it a whirl! My whole family loved it!"

by

Rebecca Feistel

1 (16 oz.) bag frozen broccoli

1 medium yellow onion, sliced

1 cup carrots, sliced

vegetable broth to sauté

1-2 teaspoons grated ginger

3-4 tablespoons Thai Brand Green Curry Paste™

1 (15 oz.) can chickpeas, drained and rinsed

1 can of unsweetened lite coconut milk

Salt, pepper or crushed red pepper to taste

4 cups cooked brown rice* (optional)

1. Put the frozen broccoli, sliced onions and carrots in a large skillet with vegetable broth and sauté for 10 minutes until starting to soften.

2. Add grated ginger and curry paste. Sauté for about 5 more minutes.

3. Add chickpeas, and coconut milk. Bring to a boil, stirring often. Lower the heat to a simmer to keep warm until ready to serve.

4. Serve over cooked brown rice or just eat it as it is. The sauce is that good!

*You can serve this over any cooked whole grain or potatoes, pasta or quinoa.

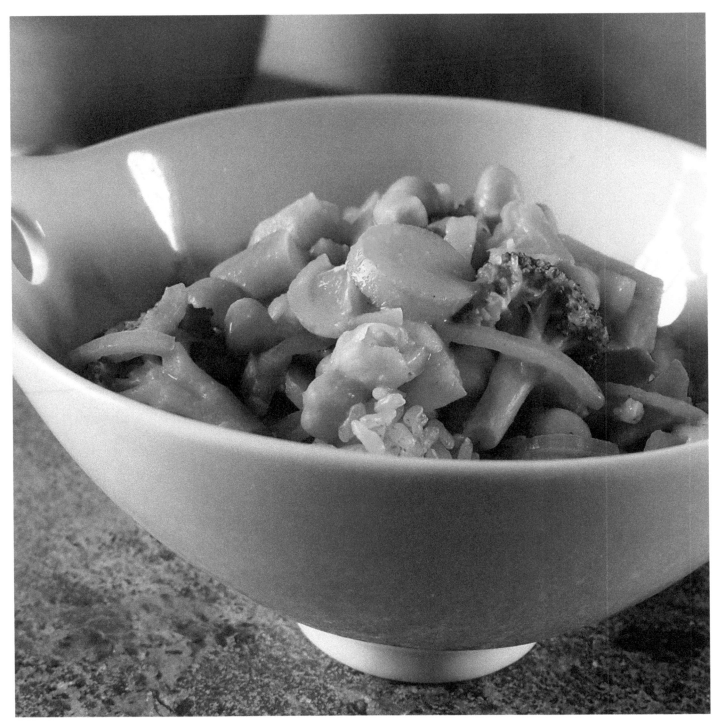

PATATAS BRAVAS

Serves 4

*This traditional Spanish dish adds a nice "kick" to
roasted potatoes*

8 yellow potatoes

FOR THE SAUCE

1 onion, thinly sliced

2 cloves garlic, minced

2 teaspoons smoked paprika

¼ tsp cayenne pepper

1 (14.5 oz.) can fire roasted tomatoes

2 teaspoons balsamic vinegar

½ tsp salt

¼ cup white wine vinegar

Fresh parsley or scallions, chopped for garnish

CASHEW GARLIC CREAM SAUCE

1 cup raw cashews, soaked 2-4 hours and drained

(If you have a high speed blender, you don't have to soak the cashews first.)

2 cloves garlic

Juice of ½ a lemon

½ cup water

1. Preheat oven to 400° F.

2. Quarter the potatoes into bite-sized chunks. Sprinkle with salt and pepper.

3. Place on a lined baking sheet and bake at 400°F for 20 minutes, flip and bake another 20 - 30 minutes until crispy.

4. While the potatoes are roasting, make the sauce.

5. Place all the sauce ingredients into a blender. Purée the sauce.

6. Pour the sauce into a small saucepan and bring to a boil then reduce to a simmer. Cook until thickened (15-20 minutes).

7. Combine cashews, garlic, lemon juice, and water in your blender and purée until very smooth.

8. When the potatoes are done, toss with the sauce. Serve with Cashew Garlic Cream Sauce sauce and chopped parsley.

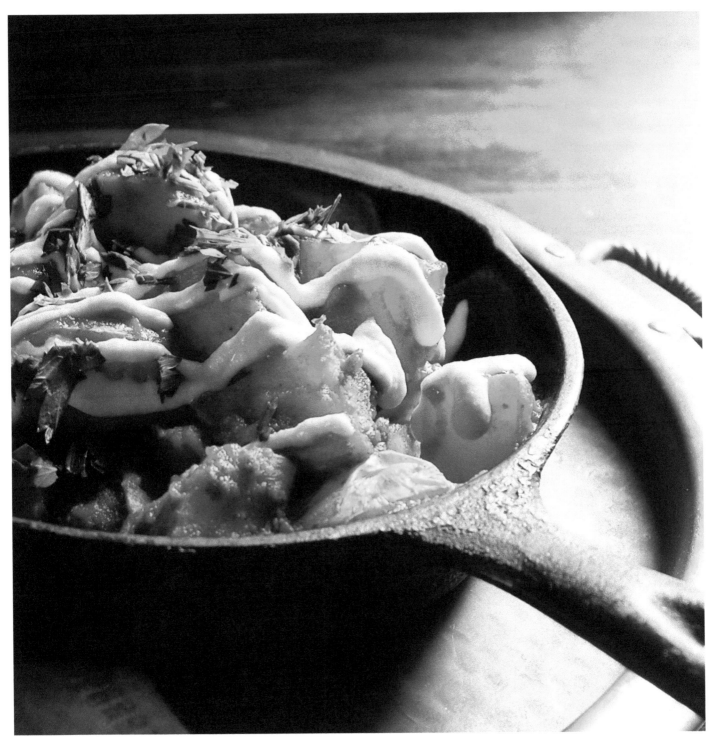

ASIAN BBQ BOWL

Serves 4

½ pkg Butler Soy Curls™ (or use tofu or tempeh)

Salt and pepper to taste

¾ cup Oil-Free BBQ Sauce (Page 94)

'Pickled' Carrots (Page 64)

Marinated Shiitake Mushrooms (Page 86)

4 cups baby spinach

4 cups cooked brown rice

1 cup edamame

3 scallions, sliced

1 cup snow peas or sliced sugar snap peas

4 tablespoons sesame seeds

Slice of lime for each bowl

1. Preheat oven to 375°F.

2. Rehydrate the soy curls in water or vegetable broth for 10 minutes.

3. Drain the soy curls and place on a lined baking sheet. Salt and pepper the soy curls. Bake for 25 minutes or until slightly crispy.

4. While soy curls are baking, make the BBQ sauce and the mushrooms.

5. Toss the soy curls in the BBQ sauce.

6. Assemble the bowl by placing 1 cup of spinach and 1 cup of rice in the bottom of a bowl and top with some soy curls, pickled carrots, edamame, scallions and pea pods. Sprinkle 1 tablespoon of sesame seeds on top.

7. Squeeze lime over each bowl before serving.

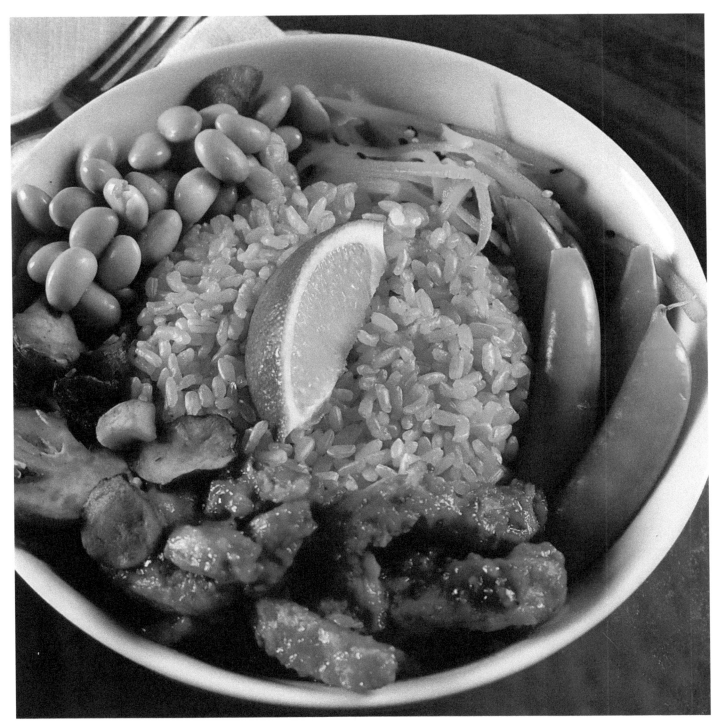

SEXY JEFFY'S SWEET POTATO CASSEROLE

Submitted by Jeffrey Hart

Serves 6

Jeff said he got the idea from a twice baked potato recipe, but he likes casseroles better than whole potatoes. This dish would be great to serve for a holiday, but it is so good and easy to make, you might want to have it other times of the year.

For the filling:

4 - 5 sweet potatoes, peeled and chopped

½ cup raisins

1 (8 oz.) can crushed pineapple

2 tablespoons maple syrup

2 tablespoons ground flax seed

1 tablespoon cinnamon

½ teaspoon nutmeg

For the topping:

1 cup of pecans, chopped

1 ½ tablespoons maple syrup

¾ cup unsweetened shredded coconut

Note: Jeff says that he sometimes substitutes apples instead of the pineapple and craisins instead of raisins. This dish is healthier than the marshmallow-topped version!

1. Preheat the oven to 375° F.

2. Boil chopped sweet potatoes until soft. Drain well.

3. Put the potatoes back in the pot and add the rest of the casserole filling ingredients and stir to combine.

4. Place the mixture into a 9 x9 glass or non-stick pan and cover with aluminum foil.

5. Bake for 20 minutes.

6. While it is baking, make the topping. On low heat in a non-stick pan, toast pecans until fragrant, stirring constantly.

7. Add the maple syrup and coconut and stir until combined. Remove from heat.

8. When the casserole is baked through, remove the tin foil. Add the topping to the casserole and bake for another 5 -10 minutes more until the topping browns a little. Serve warm.

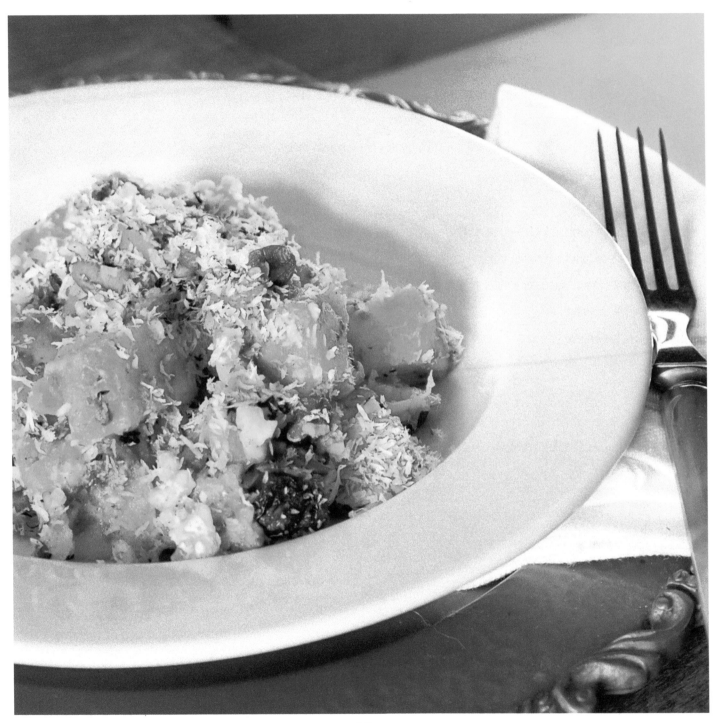

GINGERY BOK CHOY

*Bok Choy shrinks a lot when cooked. 1 pound of
bok choy serves 2 people.*

Submitted by Lynn Brown

1 pound bok choy tips or baby bok choy

2 tablespoons grated ginger root

2 large cloves fresh garlic, minced or crushed

1 - 2 tablespoons coconut aminos or tamari

Black or roasted sesame seeds or Furikake - a seaweed &
sesame sprinkle (optional)

2 cups cooked brown rice

1. Slice bok choy crosswise into ¼ to ½ inch strips. Place in large salad spinner and rinse thoroughly

2. Grate ginger on a coarse microplane zester. If you do not have a coarse zester, simply finely mince the ginger.

3. Mince or crush garlic. You can also grate on coarse microplane zester if you prefer.

4. Heat a wok to medium/high heat and add the ginger, garlic and half the greens. Stir until the ginger and garlic is mixed in.

5. As the greens begin to wilt, add remaining bok choy. There should be enough moisture on the greens that the ginger and garlic do not stick or burn. As the rest of the greens begin to wilt, drizzle with coconut aminos and continue to stir fry for approximately 2-3 minutes until the greens have wilted. The stems should still have some texture and body.

6. In a large bowl or plate, add 1 cup of rice, top with half the greens, top with sesame seeds or seaweed sprinkle (if using), and add an additional dash or two of coconut aminos to taste. Enjoy!

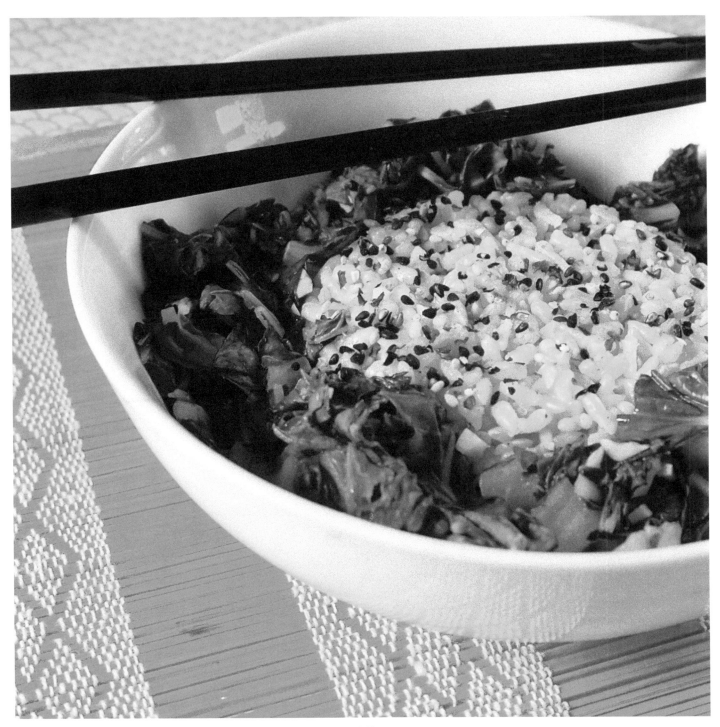

PASTA ALA VODKA

Serves 4

A much healthier version than the traditional. If you don't want to use the vodka, leave it out and replace it with vegetable broth or water. If you are allergic to nuts, replace the cashews with sunflower seeds.

1 pound whole grain pasta

1 medium onion, chopped

1 cup portobello mushrooms, sliced

1 (14.5 oz.) can diced tomatoes

1 (14.5 oz.) can fire roasted tomatoes

⅓ cup sundried tomatoes, chopped

6 cloves garlic, chopped

½ cup vodka

1 (15 oz.) can cannellini beans, drained and rinsed

½ cup raw cashews (soaked for 2 hours if you don't have a high speed blender then drained)

1 cup fresh basil, chopped

1 cup nutritional yeast

Crushed red pepper flakes to taste

Salt and pepper to taste

1. Cook pasta according to package directions.

2. While the pasta is cooking, in a medium saucepan, sauté the onion until soft.

3. Add the mushrooms and sauté until they release their liquid and the liquid evaporates.

4. Add the tomatoes and garlic. Bring to a simmer.

5. Blend the sauce with an immersion blender (or in a blender, and then return the sauce to the pot to simmer).

6. While the sauce is simmering, blend vodka, beans and cashews together.

7. Once the sauce has thickened, stir in the cashew/bean mixture and bring back to a simmer.

8. Stir in the basil and nutritional yeast.

9. Once the basil has wilted, add crushed red pepper, if desired, and season with salt and pepper.

10. Serve over pasta with a side salad and a slice of a hearty, whole grain bread.

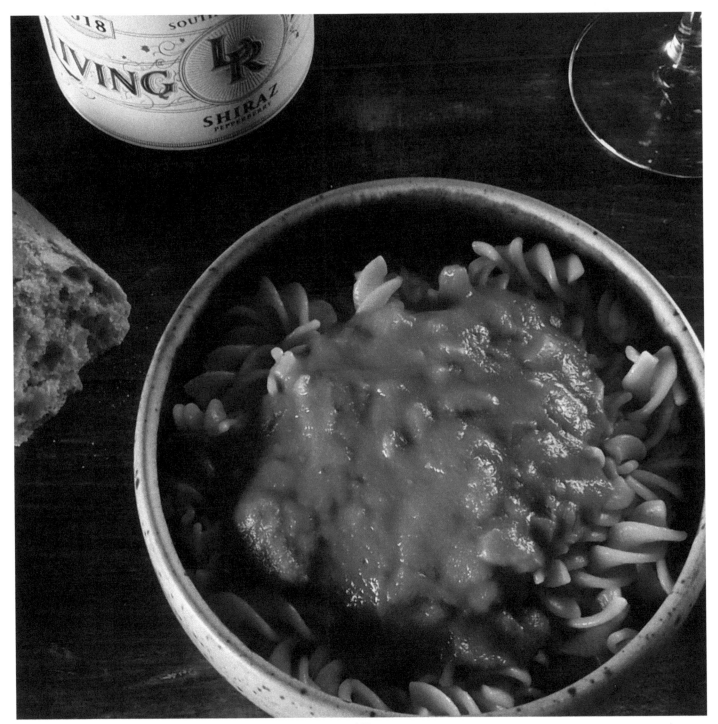

ALICE'S SPICY ORANGE GINGER STIR FRY

Serves 4–6

Alice Abrams said that she wanted to create a sauce like her favorite one from Wegmans Supermarkets. We think she succeeded. This is delicious!

¼ cup low sodium soy sauce or tamari

¾ cup orange juice

¼ cup rice vinegar

1 tablespoon fresh ginger, grated

1 clove garlic, crushed

1 - 2 tablespoons sriracha

1 ½ tablespoons cornstarch

Optional - 1 teaspoon white miso and 1 tablespoon maple syrup

4 cups stir fry vegetables of choice cut in small pieces (Carrots, onions, red peppers, shiitake mushrooms, edamame, bok choi, broccoli, snowpeas)

Optional - tempeh, tofu or soy curls

Cooked rice or noodles

1. In a small bowl, combine soy sauce, rice vinegar, orange juice, ginger, garlic, sriracha, cornstarch (and optional white miso and maple syrup to taste). Set aside.

2. Sauté stir fry vegetables, starting with carrots for 2 minutes, adding water as needed. Then add red peppers and onions and sauté for 5 minutes then add the mushrooms and saute for 3 minutes more and then add broccoli and sauté for another 3 - 5 minutes.

3. Stir in the sauce (stir well before adding). Cook to thicken, and then add snow peas (if using) and stir. Allow to sit for a few minutes so snow peas cook slightly.

4. Add tempeh, baked tofu or soy curls (if using) and serve over brown rice, golden rice or soba noodles.

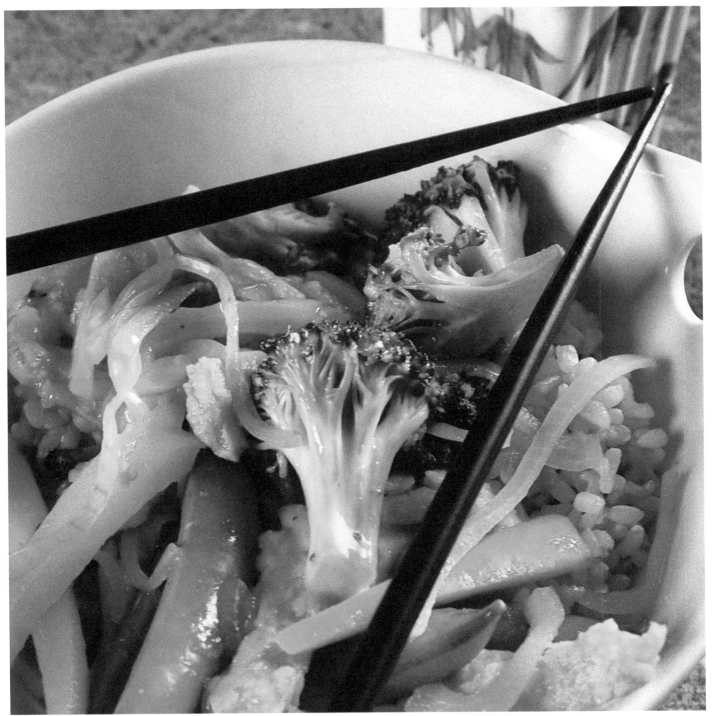

GOOD LIFE PROFILE: JEFF HART

"As a physical education teacher, health teacher, and coach I thought I had a decent concept of health. I thought the work and exercise I put in was enough, with my standard American diet, to keep me healthy and feeling well. Sure there would be down days where I feel sluggish, tired, unmotivated, and sore. I just assumed those days were normal and part of life. Weighing over 210lbs in November 2019 and having a body fat percentage of 29%, I began to feel the need to do something. I was depressed, unfit, and unmotivated. I started exercising more but I wasn't intrinsically motivated enough to maintain the intensity and frequency of the work I would need to improve. Like many people in Buffalo, NY, I would end my nights sitting at a bar with a pint of beer, ordering the meat-lover pizza and wings. I realized I needed something different.

That November, I met Doug Schmidt at a physical education and health teacher conference in NY while he was promoting the new documentary Gamechangers and his cookbook, Eat Plants Love. I had been a "poor man vegan" in college for about six months before coming home to mom-made, free, non-vegan food. Interested in the new science, I attended the session that was full of scientific evidence of the benefits of a plant-based diet. I had seen the documentary Forks Over Knives, but seeing the science finally being delivered to educators made me more confident in the information.

So I took the information for their 10-day challenge in January, not expecting to use it. I decided the day before it started to join the challenge.

After 3 days I remembered how fun cooking was again.
After 5 days my body felt like I was supercharged.
After a week I noticed a difference in my energy levels working out.

After ten days, I knew I wasn't going back to the standard American diet. In May, I stepped on the scale to reveal that I was now 169.8 lbs and 19.5% body fat. I hadn't been that fit since high school. I lost nearly 10% body fat and 40 lbs. I can't deny that I cried tears of joy. And I was happy. Life was good, cooking and eating this way. People always made it seem like eating this way is a struggle, but it's my escape. Thank you to the Schmidts for sharing their journey with me."

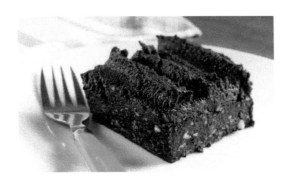

SWEET TREATS

HEARTBEET CUPCAKES

Makes 10-12

Doug created a cake for a supermarket chain years ago. In a blind taste test, his beet cake recipe won – hands down! The director of the bakery said 'I'm NOT going to sell a beet cake!' His loss, your gain! These will win your heart.

1 medium cooked beet, chopped (about ¾ cup)

½ cup maple syrup

1 teaspoon vanilla

1 ½ cups whole wheat pastry flour

¾ cup almond meal/flour

½ cup cocoa powder

2 teaspoons baking powder

1 teaspoon baking soda

½ teaspoon salt

1 cup non-dairy milk

½ cup chopped walnuts (optional)

½ cup non-dairy semi-sweet chocolate chips (optional)

We use a silicone muffin pan as it is an oil-free way of not having the muffins stick to the pan. Let cool fully before removing from pan.

1. Preheat oven to 350°F.

2. Place beet, maple syrup and vanilla in a food processor and process until combined. This doesn't have to be a purée as long as the beet is in small bits. Set aside.

3. In a medium size bowl, measure out all the dry ingredients and stir until well combined.

4. Add milk and beet purée to dry ingredients and mix until no dry ingredients are seen.

5. Add optional walnuts or chocolate chips and mix into batter.

6. Portion into silicone muffin pan (or into cupcake liners).

7. Bake at 350°F for 25-30 minutes or until a toothpick comes out clean.

8. Top with our Chocolacado Ganache on page 154.

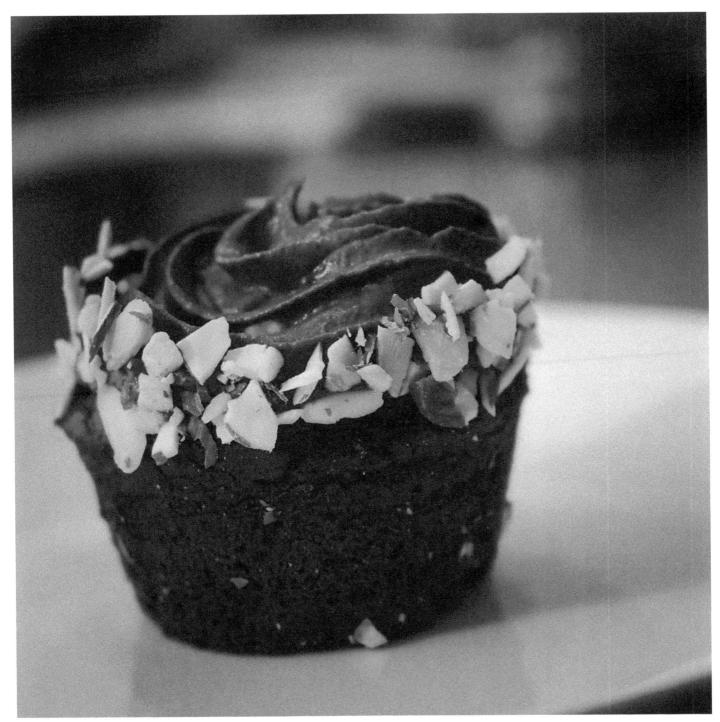

CHOCOLACADO GANACHE

Makes 1 ½ – 2 cups

1 avocado, chopped

1 (15 oz.) can black beans, drained and rinsed

6 tablespoons maple syrup

3 tablespoons dark cocoa powder

2 tablespoons cacao powder

2 tablespoons vanilla

Pinch of salt

1. Blend or purée ingredients until uniform in texture and color.
2. Refrigerate to firm for piping or until needed.

Note: You can use all dark cocoa in this if you like. It will just be darker in color.
We find that a bit of cacao adds an almost milk chocolate flavor.

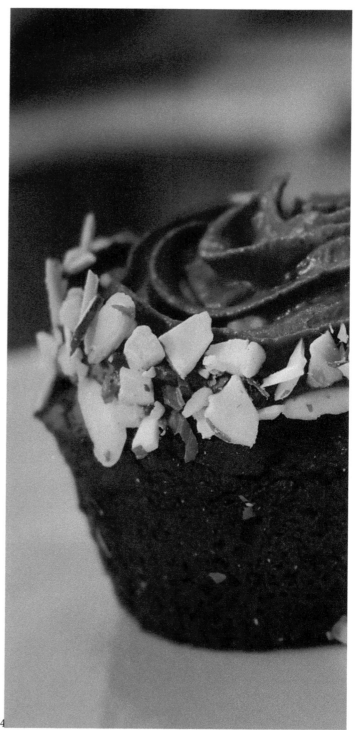

CANDIED NUTS

1 cup walnuts or pecans

½ cup maple syrup

Optional - ¼ teaspoon cinnamon

1. Place nuts and maple syrup (and cinnamon, if using) in a small saucepan.

2. Heat on high, stirring constantly to prevent burning. Cook until the maple syrup is absorbed. What you are actually doing is evaporating off any water in the maple syrup, leaving a glaze of sugar on the nuts. If properly done, the nuts will be coated in a shiny sugar glaze (this takes about 5 minutes).

3. Allow the nuts to cool on a parchment paper/ silicone lined cookie sheet. Store in a sealed container. Toss on salads.

Note: On days when humidity is high, the nuts may be a little sticky once cooled.

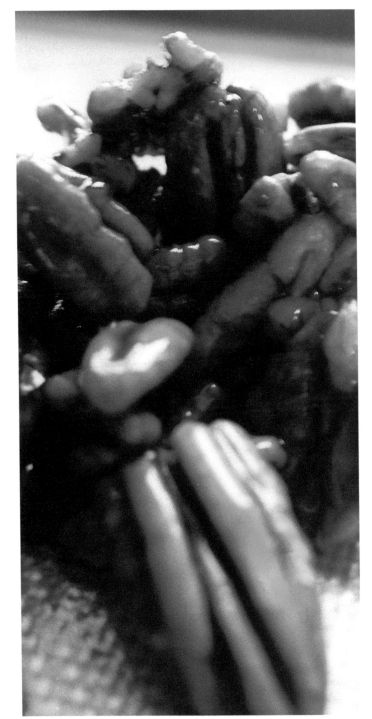

BANANAS FOSTER

Serves 3

For those times when you just need a quick,
decadent dessert.

3 bananas

½ cup chopped pecans

½ cup rolled oats

1 tablespoon rum

1 teaspoon vanilla

2 tablespoons maple syrup

1. Preheat the oven to 350° F.

2. In a shallow baking dish, place 3 bananas cut in half (not lengthwise).

3. In a food processor, pulse oats and pecans until uniform in texture.

4. In a small bowl, blend the liquid ingredients together and drizzle over the top of the bananas.

5. Sprinkle the oat/nut mixture on top of bananas.

6. Bake at 350°F for 20 minutes. Serve warm.

Note: This goes well topped with vanilla nice
cream!

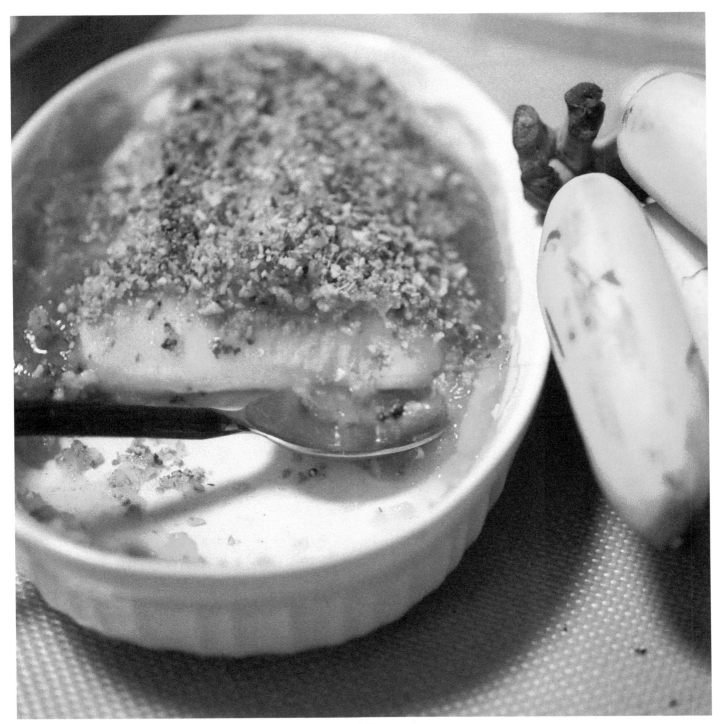

JUST PEACHY CRUMBLE

Serves 4-6

All the sweetness in this dish relies on very ripe peaches. There are no sugars added.

6 - 8 peaches, sliced

1 teaspoon almond extract

FOR THE TOPPING:

2 cups rolled oats

1 cup walnuts, chopped

1 cup almond meal/flour

1 tablespoon cinnamon

1. Preheat the oven to 375° F.

2. Slice the peaches leaving the skin on. Place them in the bottom of a 8X8 pan. Sprinkle almond extract over the top of the peaches. Mix well.

3. Take all the ingredients for the topping and pulse it in a food processor until it all comes together. Sprinkle this over the top of the peaches.

4. Bake for 45 minutes at 375° F or until nicely browned and the peaches are tender.

This goes well with vanilla nice cream.

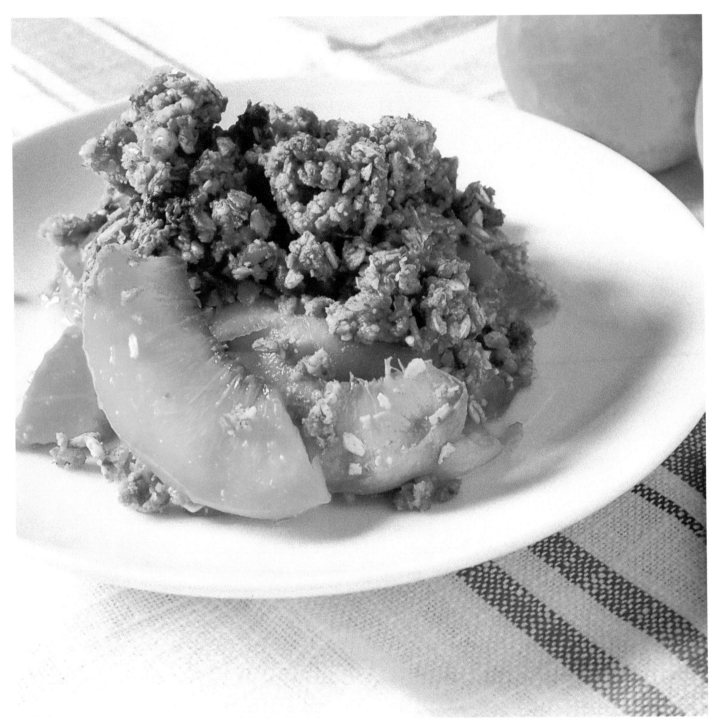

COCOA LOCO RICE BARS

Makes 12 bars

½ cup maple syrup

½ cup almond butter

½ teaspoon salt

1 teaspoon vanilla

3 cups puffed brown rice cereal

½ cup non-dairy chocolate chips

1. Place maple syrup into a sauce pan. Bring syrup to a boil.

2. Add almond butter, vanilla and salt.

3. Put the puffed brown rice and chocolate chips into a bowl.

4. Take the mixture in the pan off the heat and pour onto the rice cereal and chocolate chips. Stir until it is all coated evenly.

5. Press into the bottom of a silcone or a parchment lined 8X8 pan.

6. Chill in the refrigerator. Cut into squares and

Variations
Add dried fruits like chopped cherries, raisins, craisins, chopped
apricots or toasted coconut.
Wait until the mixture is cool and then add the chips and other
additions and the chocolate won't melt.

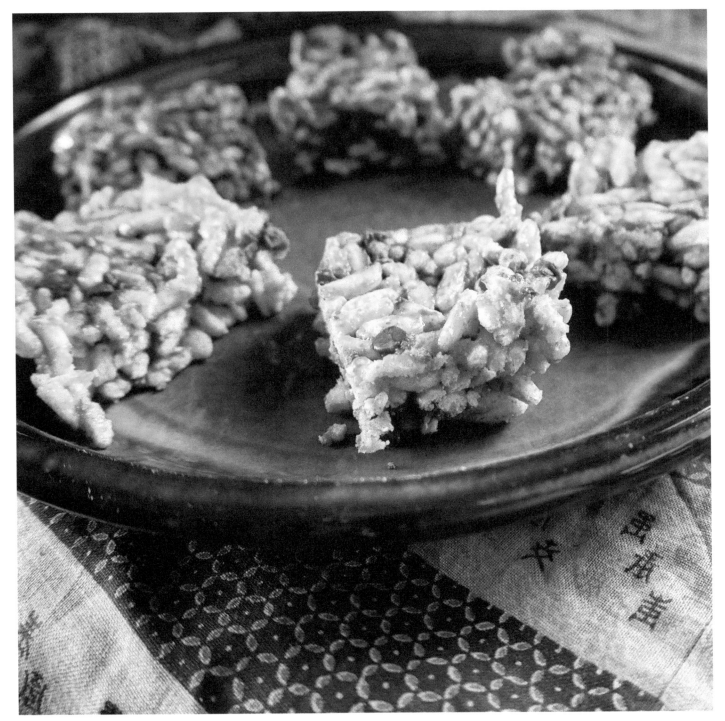

WALNUT & DATE NO-BAKE BROWNIES WITH GANACHE

Serves 12

These no-bake brownies are a favorite of our friends. They are very rich and are a rare treat. Enjoy!

2 cups walnut pieces

1 cup dark cocoa powder

1 teaspoon cinnamon

Pinch of coarse salt

2 cups Medjool dates, pitted

½ cup dried figs

1 teaspoon vanilla

1 tablespoon of Kahlúa™ (optional)

1 tablespoon maple syrup

½ cup of mini non-dairy chocolate chips

¼ cup hot water

Chocolacado Ganache (page 154)

1. In a food processor, add everything but the water, and pulse until uniform in texture and then run the food processor until it starts to come together. If it seems too dry, add ¼ cup hot water which makes a smoother texture.

2. Press into an 8x8 inch square pan (wet hands makes this easier). Set aside in the refrigerator while you make the ganache.

3. After the mixture has chilled, spread on the ganache and enjoy!

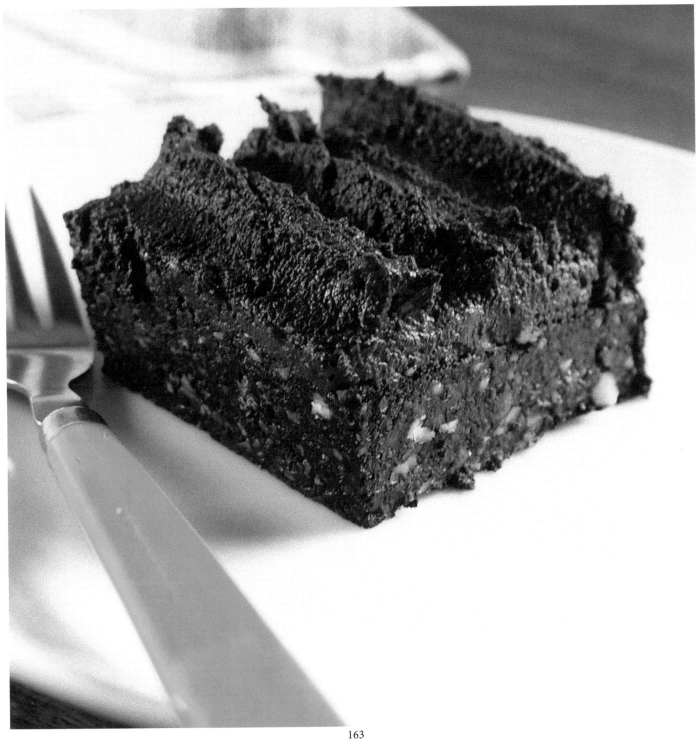

PUMPKIN SPICE CREAMER

Makes 2 ½ cups

This recipe was submitted by Darlene Cowles. Do you love everything pumpkin? Try this in your coffee for a warm autumn treat.

2 cups oat milk

7 tablespoons pumpkin purée

¼ cup maple syrup

½ teaspoon cinnamon

¼ teaspoon pumpkin spice

1. Blend everything together and keep refrigerated until ready to use.

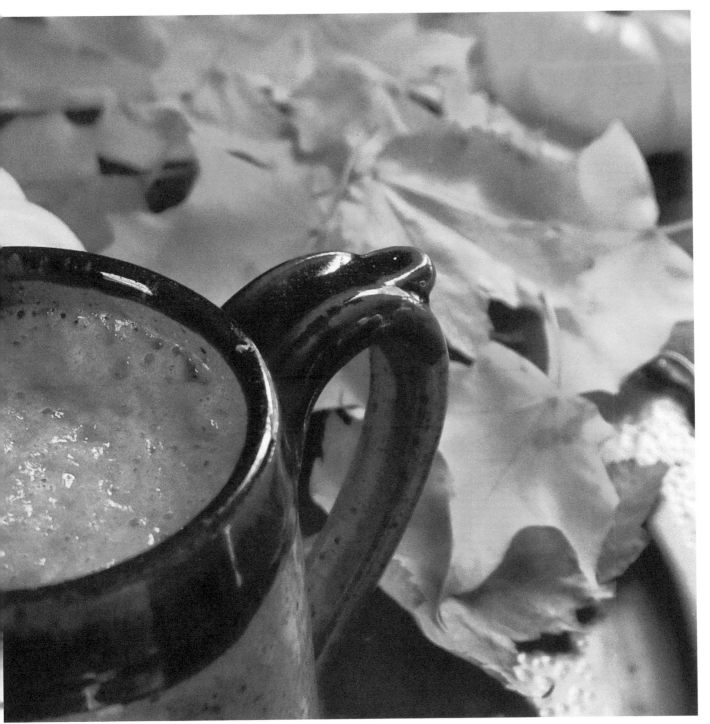

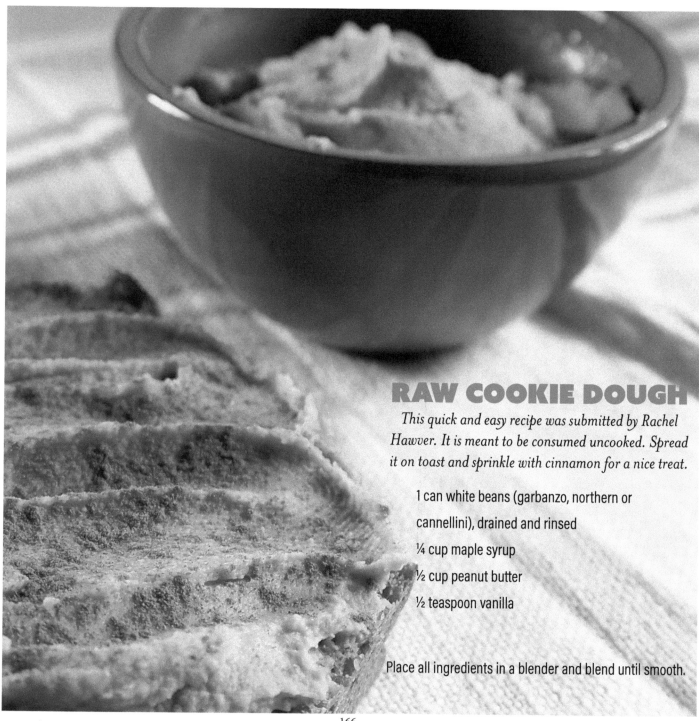

RAW COOKIE DOUGH

This quick and easy recipe was submitted by Rachel Hawver. It is meant to be consumed uncooked. Spread it on toast and sprinkle with cinnamon for a nice treat.

1 can white beans (garbanzo, northern or cannellini), drained and rinsed

¼ cup maple syrup

½ cup peanut butter

½ teaspoon vanilla

Place all ingredients in a blender and blend until smooth.

MOVING TOWARDS A PLANT-BASED DIET: INFORMATION AND RESOURCES

BOOKS TO FURTHER YOUR KNOWLEDGE

The China Study: Revised and Expanded Edition: The Most Comprehensive Study of Nutrition Ever Conducted by T. Colin Campbell and Thomas M. Campbell II

Idiot's Guide to Plant Based Nutrition 2nd Edition by Julieanna Hever and Ray Cronise

How Not to Die: Discover the Foods Scientifically Proven to Prevent and Reverse Disease by Michael Greger MD

The China Study Solution: The Simple Way to Lose Weight and Reverse Illness, Using a Whole-Food, Plant-Based Diet by Thomas Campbell

Prevent and Reverse Heart Disease: The Revolutionary, Scientifically Proven, Nutrition-Based Cure by Caldwell B. Esselstyn Jr. M.D.

The Healthiest Diet on the Planet: Why the Foods You Love - Pizza, Pancakes, Potatoes, Pasta, and More - Are the Solution to Preventing Disease by John McDougall

The Forks Over Knives Plan: How to Transition to the Life-Saving, Whole-Food, Plant-Based Diet by Alona Pulde and Matthew Lederman

Dr. Neal Barnard's Program for Reversing Diabetes: The Scientifically Proven System for Reversing Diabetes without Drugs by Neal D. Barnard and Bryanna Clark Grogan

Proteinaholic: How Our Obsession with Meat Is Killing Us and What We Can Do About It
by Garth Davis M.D. and Howard Jacobson

The Engine 2 Seven-Day Rescue Diet: Eat Plants, Lose Weight, Save Your Health By Rip Esselstyn

The Healthspan Solution: How and What to Eat to Add Life to Your Years by Raymond J. Cronise, Julieanna Hever M.S., R.D.

The Plant-Based Solution - America's Healthy Heart Doc's Plan to Power Your Health by Joel K. Kahn, MD

The Alzheimer's Solution: A Breakthrough Program to Prevent and Reverse the Symptoms of Cognitive Decline at Every Age by Dean and Ayesha Sherzai MD

Eat to Live: The Amazing Nutrient-Rich Program for Fast and Sustained Weight Loss by Joel Fuhrman MD

COOKBOOKS

Plant Pure Nation Cookbook by Kim Campbell

The Prevent and Reverse Heart Disease Cookbook: Over 125 Delicious, Life-Changing, Plant-Based Recipes by Ann Crile Esselstyn and Jane Esselstyn

Perfectly Plant-Based Recipe Book by PBNSG

The Plantpower Way: Whole Food Plant-Based Recipes and Guidance for The Whole Family by Rich Roll, Julie Piatt

Plant-Powered Families: Over 100 Kid-Tested, Whole-Foods Vegan Recipes by Dreena Burton

Forks Over Knives Family: Every Parent's Guide to Raising Healthy, Happy Kids on a Whole-Food, Plant-Based Diet by Alona Pulde and Matthew Lederman M.D.

The Help Yourself Cookbook for Kids: 60 Easy Plant-Based Recipes Kids Can Make to Stay Healthy and Save the Earth by Ruby Roth

The China Study Cookbook: Over 120 Whole Food, Plant-Based Recipes
by LeAnne Campbell and T. Colin Campbell

The How Not To Die Cookbook by Dr. Micheal Greger and recipes by Robin Robertson

Plant Pure Kitchen by Kim Campbell

The Vegiterranean Diet: The New and Improved Mediterranean Eating Plan -by Julieanna Hever

The Vegan 8 by Brandi Doming

MOVIES

Forks Over Knives

The Gamechangers

PlantPure Nation

Cowspiracy

The Kids Menu

Eating You Alive

What the Health

IMMERSIONS AND LIVE-IN PROGRAMS

Dr. John McDougall's Programs https://www.drmcdougall.com/health/programs/

Engine 2 Events/Immersions https://2forksevents.com/

True North Health Center https://www.healthpromoting.com/

Dr. Joel Fuhrman's Eat To Live Retreats https://www.drfuhrman.com/etlretreat

USEFUL WEBSITES

http://www.dresselstyn.com/

Dr. Caldwell Esselstyn's site talking about preventing and reversing heart disease

http://nutritionfacts.org/

Dr. Michael Greger's site which scours the medical journals for the latest research and makes it accessible to the layman. If you have a health question you can usually find a reference here. No hype or industry marketing just the facts.

https://www.forksoverknives.com

A site with inspirational stories, recipes and more to help you get on your way.

https://www.pbnsg.org/

Plant Based Nutrition Support Group is a non-profit organization dedicated to evidence-based education and advocacy of plant-based whole food nutrition and an active lifestyle, to help you prevent or reverse chronic disease and achieve optimal health.

https://plantbasednetwork.com/

Plant Based Network officially launched on Nov 1st (World Vegan Day) in Charlotte, NC, as a lifestyle and entertainment media company that promotes plant-based living.

https://plantbaseddietitian.com/about/

Registered Dietitian Julieanna Hever's site. She has clients the world over.

https://engine2diet.com/

Dr. Caldwell Esselstyn's son, Rip Esselstyn, firefighter and triathlete, promotes the Engine 2 Diet. The site has recipes and advice to get you started.

http://www.pcrm.org/

The Physicians Committee is leading a revolution in medicine.

https://masteringdiabetes.org/

Get control of your diabetes.

https://goodbyelupus.com/

Eat plants to heal your autoimmune diseases with Dr. Brooke Goldner

https://www.paddisonprogram.com/

Heal your rheumatoid arthritis with Clint Paddison

https://www.healthyhumanrevolution.com/

Healthy Human Revolution

https://eatplantslove.com/

Eat Plants Love

https://fatmanrants.com/

Fatmanrants with Tim and Heather Kaufman

https://www.theliftproject.global/

The Lift Project with Dr. Darren Morton

https://www.chrisbeatcancer.com/

Learn how to beat cancer with Chris Wark

https://www.drmcdougall.com/

Follow Dr. John McDougall's starch based diet.

PODCASTS AND YOUTUBE CHANNELS

The Rich Roll Podcast - https://www.richroll.com/category/podcast/

Plant Strong Podcast https://www.plantstrongpodcast.com/

Brain Health and Beyond with Team Sherzai

https://podcasts.apple.com/us/podcast/brain-health-and-beyond-with-team-sherzai-md/id1474018356

Feel Better, Live More with Dr. Rangan Chatterjee

https://podcasts.apple.com/us/podcast/feel-better-live-more-with-dr-rangan-chatterjee/id1333552422

Nutrition Facts with Dr. Greger

https://podcasts.apple.com/us/podcast/nutrition-facts-with-dr-greger/id1183093544

Eat Plants Love Youtube https://www.youtube.com/channel/UC18PgLNRZuRvDTBQ5opQ46g

The Jaroudi Family Youtube Channel

https://www.youtube.com/channel/UCOQJr9oAj3iu4ig3r08fm-Q

Krocks in the Kitchen Youtube Channel

https://www.youtube.com/channel/UC9vlrPTF0znhis-gsFB8l8Q

The PlantYourself Podcast - http://plantyourself.com/category/podcast/

Nutritionfacts.org podcast - https://nutritionfacts.org/video-podcast-subscribe/

Chef AJ's Youtube Channel - https://www.youtube.com/channel/UCDHK7RywWc4z8J5K3MKkvRw

Jane Esselstyn's Youtube Channel -https://www.youtube.com/channel/UCkVtuE3WR0NhNnDiP5d_pAA

Jill McKeever's Fun Youtube Channel - https://www.youtube.com/channel/UCzreeLY8gsp8NoqhG9OnqIQ

RECIPE BLOGGERS

The Vegan 8 with Brandi Doming - https://thevegan8.com/

Brand New Vegan with Chuck Underwood - https://www.brandnewvegan.com/

The Fatfree Vegan with Susan Voisin - https://fatfreevegan.com/

Straight Up Food with Cathy Fisher - https://www.straightupfood.com/blog/

Plantiful Kiki - https://plantifulkiki.com/

Monkey and Me Kitchen Adventures - https://monkeyandmekitchenadventures.com/

APPS

Greger's Daily Dozen

Plant Based Networks

Vanilla Bean

The Beet

Forks Over Knives

Happy Cow

Oh She Glows

PCRM'S Nutrition Guide

WHOLE PLANT FOOD BASIC PANTRY

You do not have to purchase everything on this list and there are many other foods that you can add to your pantry. Soon you will find what you use the most to keep your own pantry stocked. This is just a suggested list of the basic items you could purchase to get started.

LEGUMES (CAN OR DRIED)

Black beans
Lentils
Chickpeas
White (navy, northern or cannellini) beans
Pinto beans
Kidney beans
Fat free refried beans
Split peas

GRAINS

Quinoa
Brown rice
Rolled Oats
Oat Groats
Bulgur
Wheat berries
Farro
Barley
Whole grain pasta

SPICES

Oregano
Rosemary
Thyme
Dried chili flakes
Curry powder
Cumin
Coriander
Garlic powder
Onion powder
Cinnamon
Nutmeg
Cloves
Smoked paprika
Ground ginger
Turmeric
Black Cumin

VINEGARS AND CONDIMENTS

Raw apple cider vinegar
Flavored Balsamic vinegars
Rice vinegar
Red and/or white vinegar
Low sodium soy sauce and/or
Low sodium tamari
Coconut aminos
Dijon mustard
Ketchup (no high fructose corn syrup)
Hot sauce
Nut butters
Almond butter (no added oil)
Peanut butter (no added oil)
Tahini (Sesame Paste)

Sweeteners
Maple syrup
Date sugar
Brown rice syrup
Seeds
Chia seeds
Flax seeds
Hemp seeds
Sesame seeds
Sunflower seeds

SHELF STABLE UNSWEETENED PLANT MILKS (CHOOSE ALL OR SOME)

Almond
Soy
Oat
Hemp
Rice

MISCELLANEOUS

Butler Soy Curls™
Whole wheat panko crumbs
Chickpea crumbs
Raw cacao nibs or non-dairy chocolate chips
Cocoa powder
Low sodium Vegetable broth
Nutritional yeast (NOOCH)
Vanilla extract
Almond extract

FLOURS

Whole wheat flour
Chickpea flour
Oat flour
Corn flour/meal

DRIED FRUITS AND NUTS

Raisins
Dates
Figs
Nuts
Walnuts
Brazil nuts
Raw cashews
Almonds

CANNED AND BOTTLED GOODS

Canned tomatoes
Tomato paste
Mustard
Salsa

BULBS AND ROOTS

Sweet potatoes
White potatoes
Onions
Garlic

PRODUCE AND REFRIGERATOR ITEMS

This can vary widely depending on your tastes. We find that if we have these basic items, (and the pantry items) we can easily throw together a meal in minutes.

PLANT BASED MILKS (ANY OR ALL)

Almond
Soy
Oat
Rice

VEGETABLES

Kale
Broccoli
Lettuce
Spinach
Red Peppers
Carrots
Cucumbers
Brussels sprouts
Beets
Scallions/Green onions

FRUITS

All kinds of berries
Bananas
Apples
Oranges
Lemons
Any seasonal fruit

MISCELLANEOUS

Applesauce
Miso
Tofu
Tempeh
Sauerkraut
Mushrooms

Index

CPSIA information can be obtained
at www.ICGtesting.com
Printed in the USA
BVHW020113201220
596042BV00002B/5